MW01640357

To A Very Dear Frie[illegible]
Mike.

You're a great friend.
Looking foward to many
great times.

Elliot Rand "D.D.S."!!

To Be with
God's help!!

Complete and Anchored Dentures

Jack M. Buchman, D.D.S., F.I.C.D., F.A.G.D., F.A.C.P.

Postgraduate Visiting Prosthetic Instructor at Tufts University School of Dental Medicine and University of Pittsburgh School of Dental Medicine

Chief of Prosthetics, Israel Dental Association, Haifa Branch

Overseas Director, Haifa Institute for Advanced Dental Education

Chief Consultant of Complete Denture Prosthesis, Tel Aviv University, Sackler School of Medicine, School of Continuing Medical Education, Dental Division, Ramat-Aviv, Israel

Ajax Menekratis, D.D.S., F.I.C.D.

Docteur en Chirurgie Dentaire. Paris, France.

Member of the National Academy of Dental Surgery, France
Member of the American Dental Society of Europe

Fellow of the Society of Oral Physiology and Occlusion

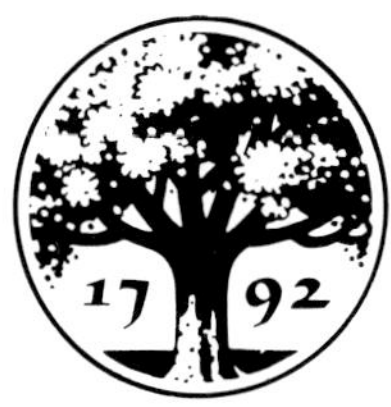

J. B. Lippincott Company
Philadelphia • Toronto

ISBN 0-397-50336-9

Library of Congress Catalog Card Number 74-2236

Printed in the United States of America

1 3 5 4 2

Library of Congress Cataloging in Publication Data

Buchman, Jack M

Complete and anchored dentures.

1. Complete dentures. I. Menekratis, Ajax, joint author. II. Title. [DNLM: 1. Denture, Complete—Atlases. 2. Denture, Partial, Fixed—Atlases. WU17 B919c 1974]

RK655.B8 617.6'92 74-2236

ISBN 0-397-50336-9

Foreword

I am most flattered that Dr. Jack Buchman, whom I deeply respect for his contributions to the development of prosthodontics and gnathology, has given me the opportunity to write a Foreword to this work.

I am greatly indebted to Jack Buchman for what he has taught me, as I am also indebted to other enthusiastic and creative practitioners—Drs. Beverly B. McCollum, Harvey Stallard, Charles E. Stuart, Gian Carlo Chiarini, Sumiya Hobo, Donald MacQueen, David McLean, Mario Martignoni, Claude Nabors, Olympio Pinto, Ulf Posselt, Carlos Ripol and Alfred Steiger.

The word gnathology was coined by Dr. Beverly B. McCollum and Dr. Harvey Stallard and pertains to the study of the masticatory apparatus as a biologic unit as well as tooth morphology, anatomy, histology, physiology, pathology, the therapeutics of the oral cavity, with emphasis on the jaws and teeth and the vital relations of this organ to the rest of the body.

Sound reconstruction is impossible without an appreciation of gnathology and an understanding of the science of occlusion. Nevertheless, despite their importance, both subjects remain among the most challenging and most discussed fields in dentistry. A thorough background in the fundamentals of dental anatomy and the physiology of occlusal function and dysfunction is absolutely necessary. Consequently, we should dedicate ourselves, as Drs. Buchman and Menekratis have, to patient, knowledgeable diagnosis and unhurried technique—keeping in mind the ultimate objective of the health and well-being of our patients.

PETER K. THOMAS, B.Sc., D.D.S.
Beverly Hills, California

Preface

In this book we have tried to present a detailed, concise description of the construction of the complete denture for the non-problem case seen in every dentist's office. Part I sets forth in a minimal amount of text, and a maximal number of full-color illustrations, the steps required to fabricate a complete denture that will be pleasing and satisfactory in both form and function. The reconstructive procedures described are both a simplification and an extension of those in AN ATLAS OF COMPLETE DENTURE PROSTHESIS (Lippincott; 1970), techniques that have proved effective after decades of rewarding but often frustrating study, experimentation and practice.

In Part II, my colleague, Dr. Ajax Menekratis, has, on the basis of my full denture techniques, developed a uniquely effective, functionally sound, and clinically proven anchored denture technique (combined with a variety of attachments, root treatment and gingivectomy, and in some cases alveolectomy).

These two techniques give the dentist a superior method of procedure regardless of whether the patient has lost all his teeth, or is still in possession of teeth that cannot be used for fixed bridgework because of bone resorption and mobility. The techniques are presented step-by-step in numerical order, to help all dentists adopt and practice them.

With humility and gratitude to our many teachers and colleagues, we are convinced that this atlas offers the dentist a comprehensive technique for sound and effective reconstruction which, when carefully executed, will satisfy in terms of esthetics, function and comfort, the high standards of modern dentistry.

JACK M. BUCHMAN

Contents

Part I: Complete Dentures

Part II: Anchored Dentures

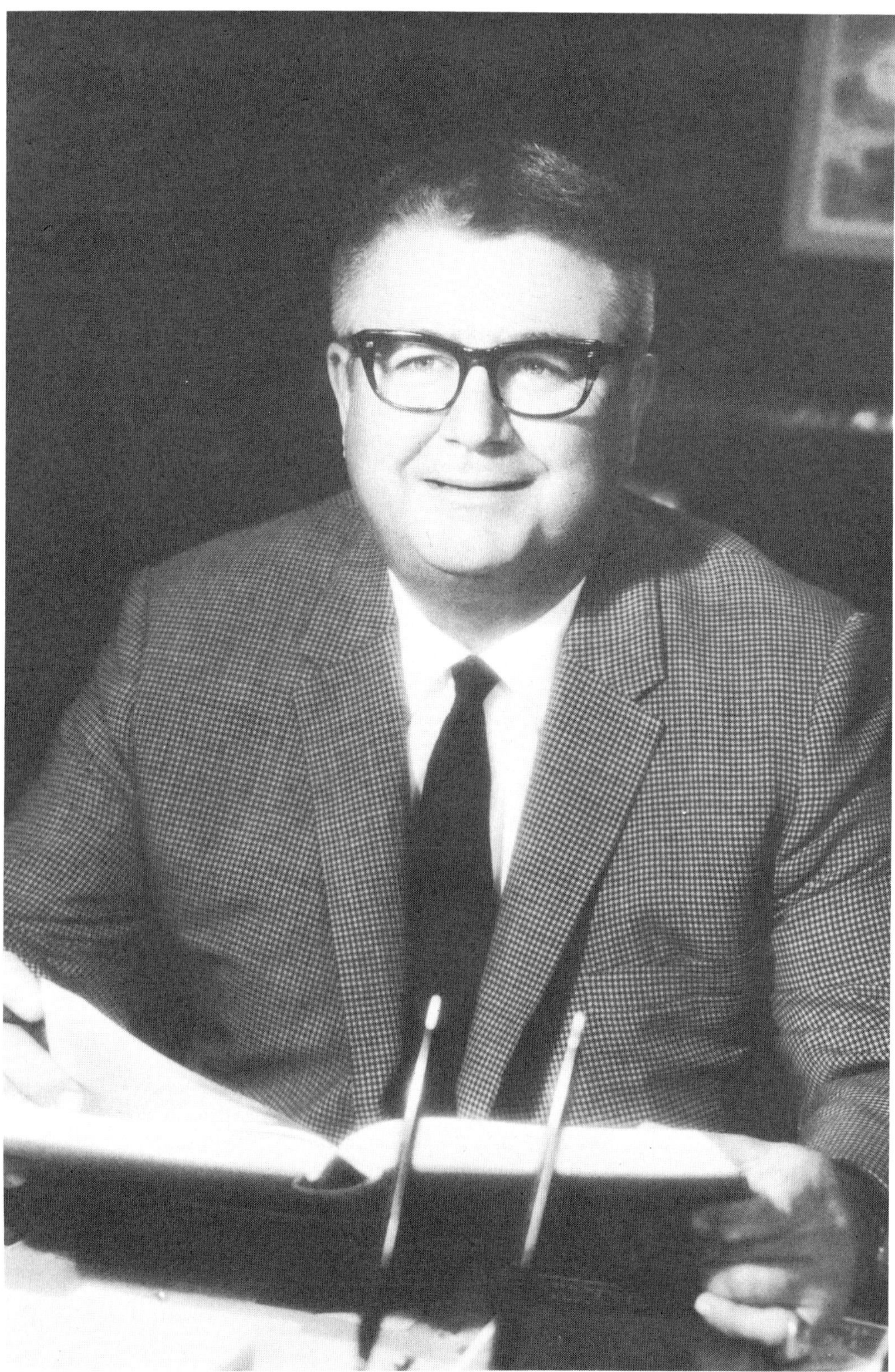

With pride and pleasure I dedicate this book to my dear friend and teacher, and one of the world's great dental practitioners, Dr. Peter K. Thomas.

PART I

Complete Dentures

Jack M. Buchman, D.D.S., F.I.C.D., F.A.G.D.

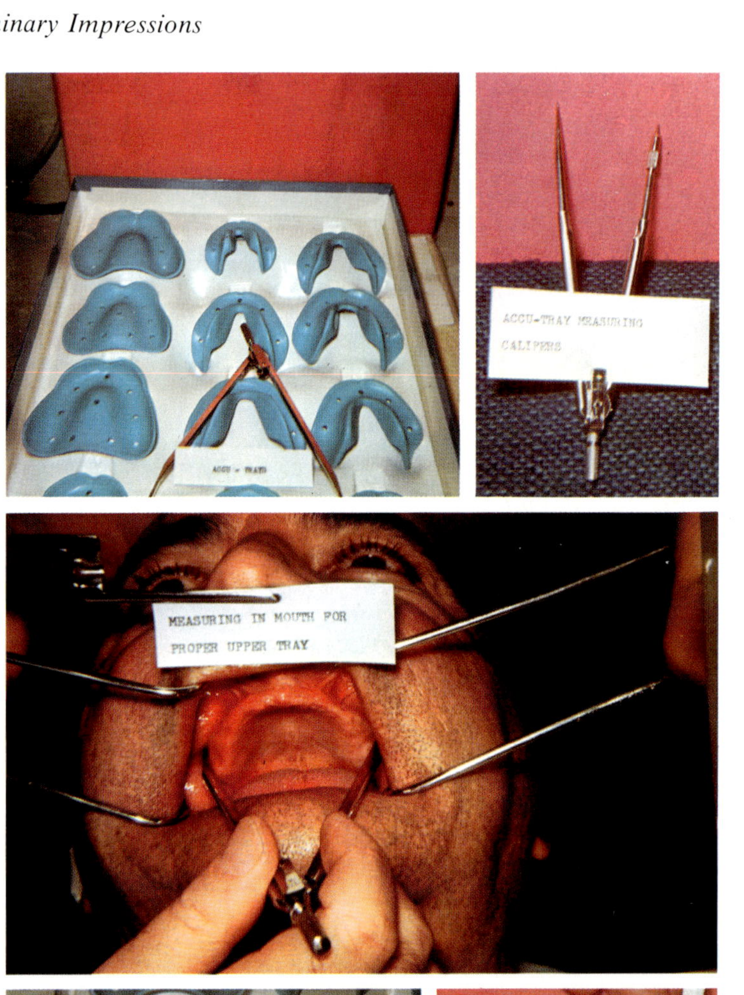

Fig. 1-1

Fig. 1-2

Fig. 1-3

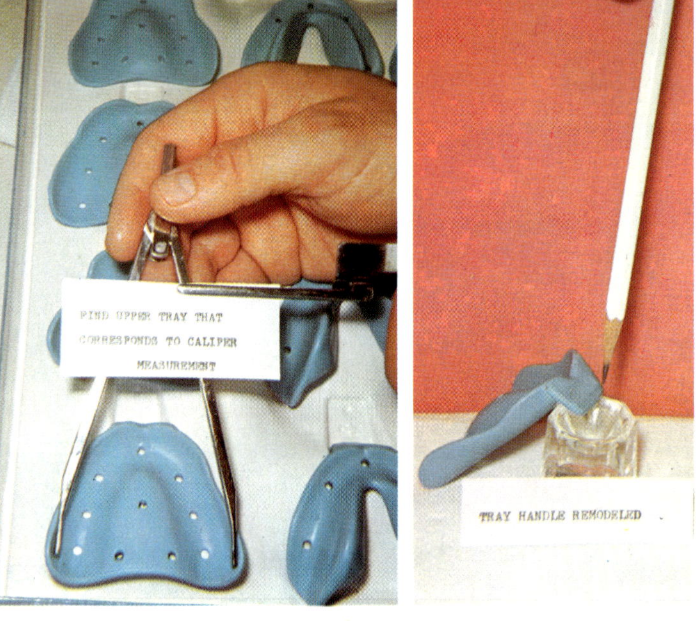

Fig. 1-4

Fig. 1-5

1. Preliminary Impressions

After thorough consultation with the patient, and evaluation of the denture problem, we proceed to the taking of preliminary impressions.

PRELIMINARY UPPER IMPRESSIONS

Dentists may be tempted to take a quick snap impression and later correct the imperfections of this snap impression during the taking of the wash impression. This should never be done. It is essential to take as accurate a preliminary impression as possible, because if the preliminary impression is inaccurate it is difficult to take a good wash impression.

1. Using the Accu-Tray kit* (Fig. 1-1), or an equivalent set-up, and the measuring calipers (Fig. 1-2):
2. Measure in the patient's mouth the distance between the buccal aspect of the maxilla in the region of the third molar on one side to the same point on the opposite side (Fig. 1-3). The measurement is always taken at the widest part of the maxilla. This affords the selection of a tray (Fig. 1-4) that will fit better from buccal to buccal than a tray selected arbitrarily.
3. Try the tray of choice in the mouth to verify the fit. Remodel the handle on the tray (Fig. 1-5).

*Accu-Tray Kit. John Lust, Bonvini Dental Laboratory, 4695 Main Street, Bridgeport, Conn. 06606

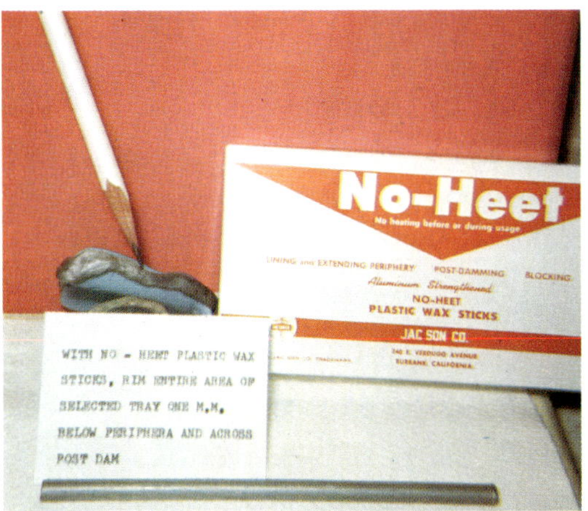

Fig. 1-6

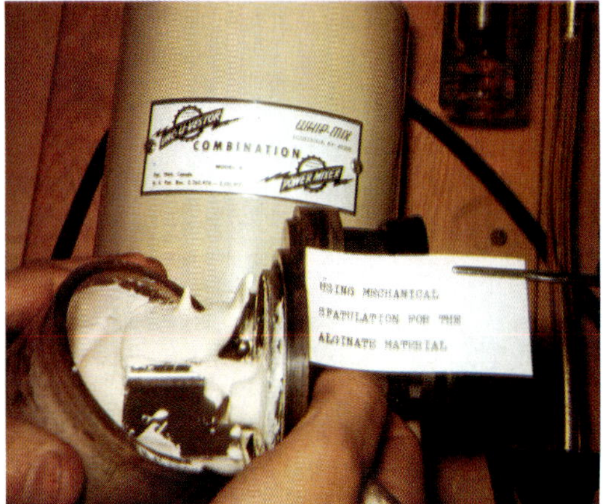

Fig. 1-7

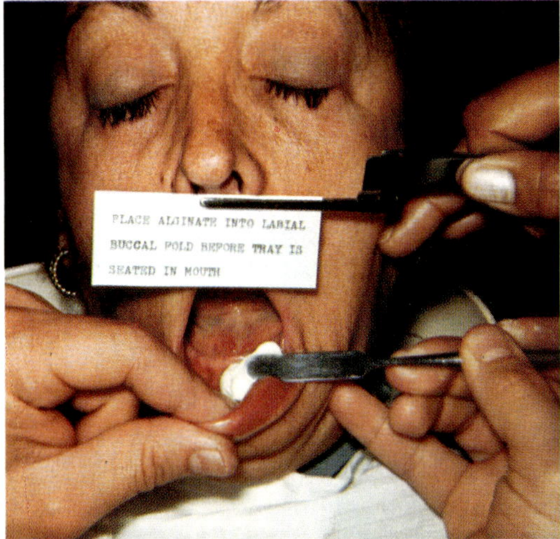

Fig. 1-8

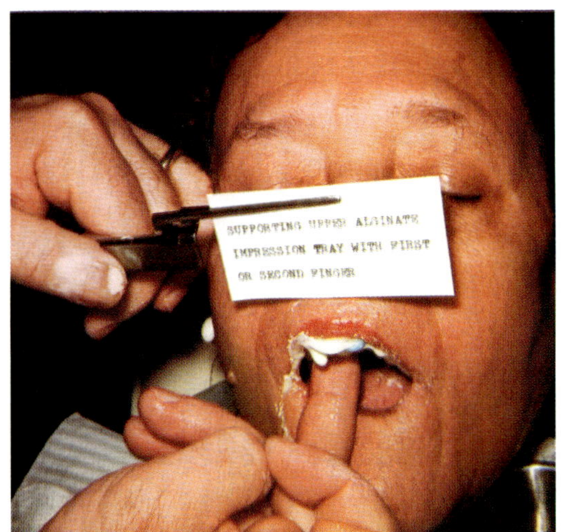

Fig. 1-9

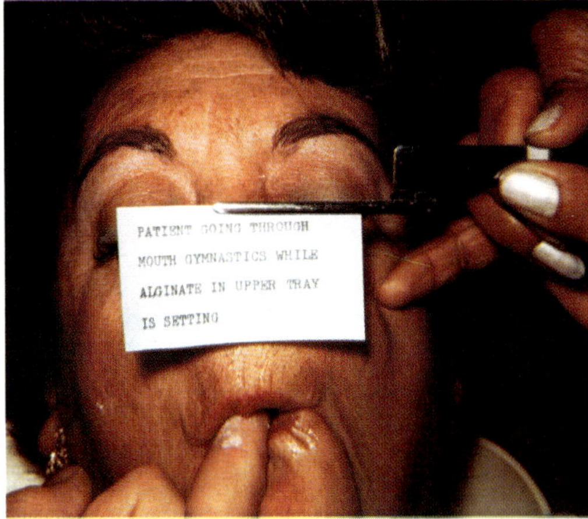

Fig. 1-10

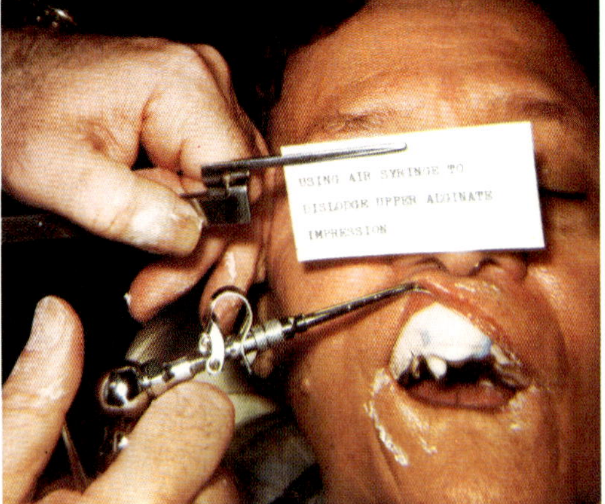

Fig. 1-11

A. Place No-Heet* plastic wax sticks (reducing the thickness of the wax somewhat) 0.5 mm. below the entire periphery and across the post-dam of the upper tray (Fig. 1-6).
B. Insert this wax-rimmed tray in the mouth and have the patient go through mouth gymnastics.
C. Remove the rimmed tray from the mouth to take an alginate impression.

4. For impression material I prefer Fast Set Alginate.†After shaking the alginate in the can thoroughly, measure out two full scoops into a rubber bowl, add 30 cc. of tap water, mix this mass either by using a heavy spatula or—better yet—by using a Whip-Mix mechanical spatulator (Fig. 1-7) set to spatulate for one minute.

5. Remove the alginate from the bowl with a spatula and place it in the tray selected.

6. Just before placing the tray in the mouth, with your fingers place some of the left-over alginate in the anterior and posterior buccal corridors of the mouth (Fig. 1-8).

7. The patient is asked to open his mouth wide to permit the introduction of the loaded tray, and once the tray has been introduced he is asked to close his mouth half way. The tray is then seated in place with a vibrating motion and held lightly in place by the operator's first or second finger on the roof of the tray (Fig. 1-9).

8. The patient is instructed immediately to go through facial gymnastics (Fig. 1-10), the motions of kissing, grinning and moving the mandible from side to side.

9. The last step—having the patient move the mandible from side to side—allows the coronoid process of the mandible to establish the preliminary thickness of the buccal border of the upper denture in the region that comes in contact during this lateral movement. (In many instances this step is overlooked, which may be a cause of subsequent dislodgement of the upper denture during function.)

10. After 5 minutes remove the upper preliminary impression by having the patient balloon the cheeks out and blow, or use an air syringe (Fig. 1-11).

11. To avoid distortion of the alginate impression, pour up this impression immediately, using any good stone composition. Invert the poured impression with the stone up, which prevents the stone from falling away from the impression. (Boxing the impression is not necessary.) Separate the stone cast from the impression.

---

*No-Heet Plastic Wax Sticks. Jac Son Co. 3416 Victory Blvd., Burbank, Calif.

†Normal Alginate. The L. D. Caulk Co., Milford, Del. 19963

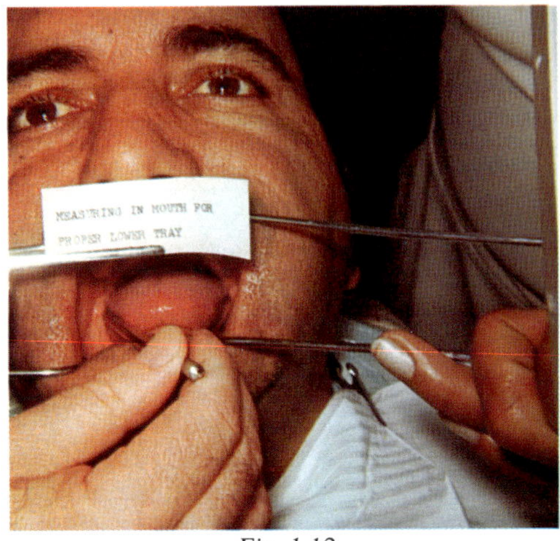

Fig. 1-12

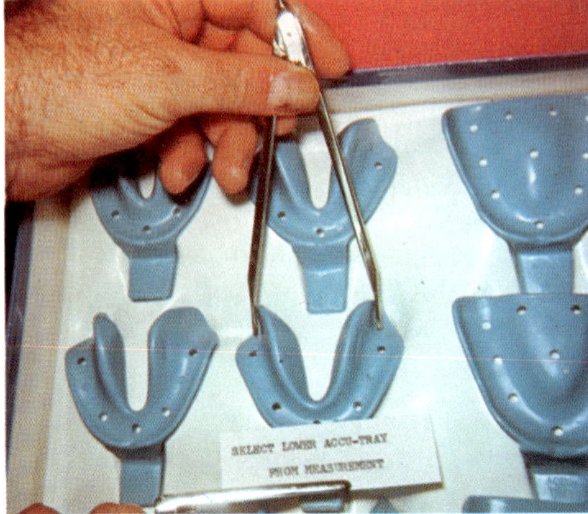

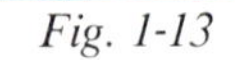

Fig. 1-13

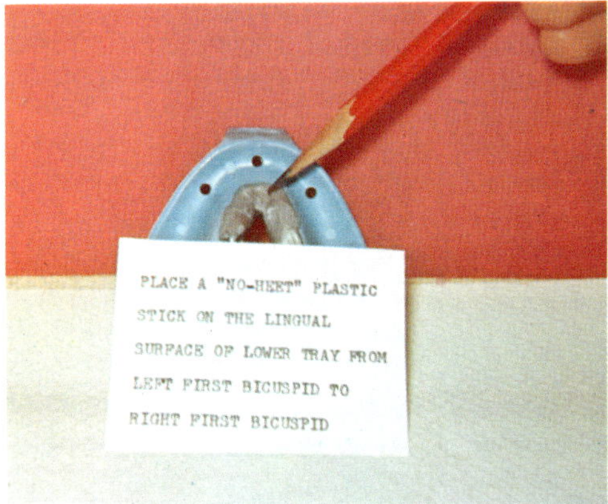

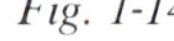

Fig. 1-14

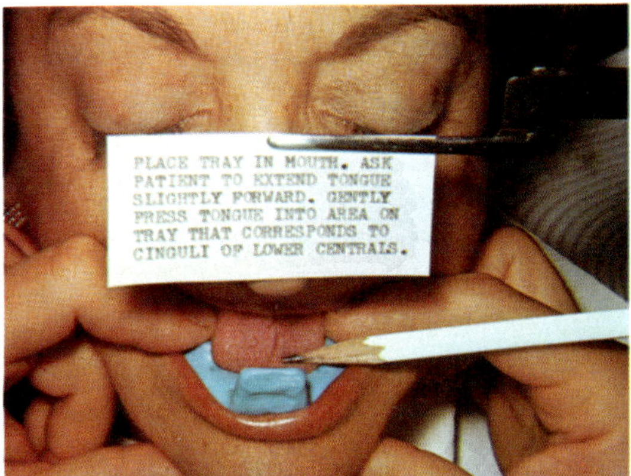

Fig. 1-15

PRELIMINARY LOWER IMPRESSIONS

1. With the calipers, measure the space between the lingual aspect of the retromolar pad on one side of the mouth to the same point on the other side of the mouth (Fig. 1-12).

2. Select an acrylic tray of proper width, as determined with the calipers (Fig. 1-13). Always measure the tray from the lingual aspect, as was done in the mouth.

3. Try the tray of choice in the mouth to verify the fit. Remodel the handle as was done in step 3A for upper impressions.

   A. Place a No-Heet plastic wax stick on the sublingual aspect from the first bicuspid on one side to the first bicuspid on opposite side (Fig. 1-14).

4. Insert this tray, with the wax on the sublingual aspect, and have the patient push his tongue slightly forward against the area of cinguli of the lower central incisors (Fig. 1-15) while you steady the tray with the fingers of both hands.

5. Remove the tray from the mouth and air dry it thoroughly. With somewhat thinned out No-Heet plastic wax sticks, rim the remaining part of the tray 0.5

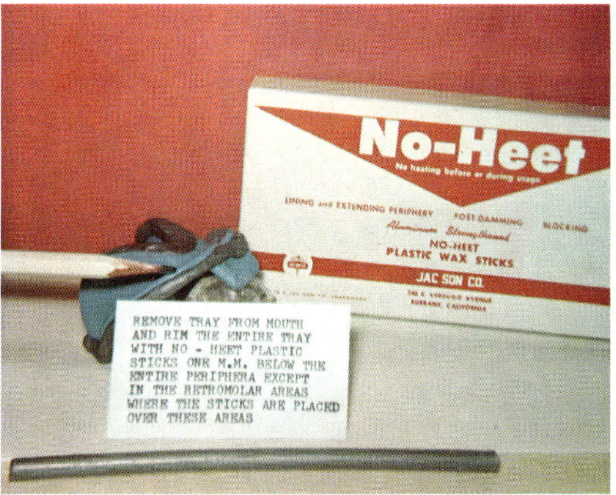

Fig. 1-16

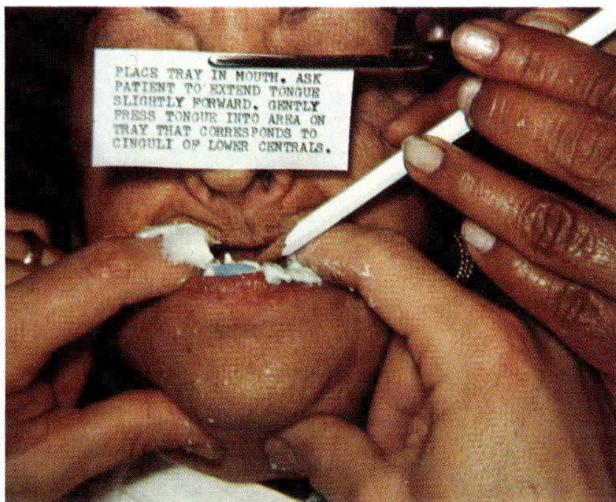

Fig. 1-17

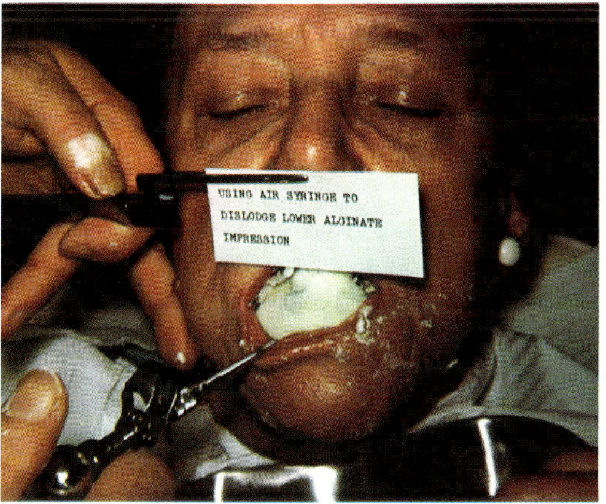

Fig. 1-18

STONE POURED ALGINATE
IMPRESSIONS PLACED IN
UPRIGHT POSITION UNTIL
STONE SETS

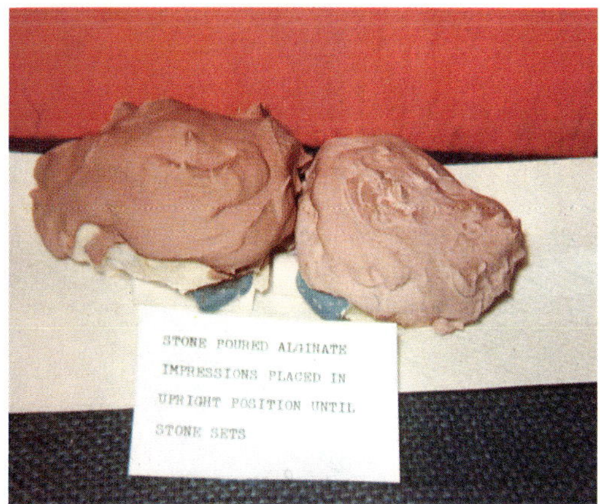

Fig. 1-19

mm. below the entire periphery (Fig. 1-16).

6. Insert this wax-rimmed tray in the mouth and, while steadying the tray with the fingers of both hands, ask the patient to go through the mouth gymnastics of puckering, grinning and opening wide.

7. Remove the rimmed tray from the mouth to take an alginate impression.

8. Follow steps 4 through 7.

9. The patient is immediately instructed to lightly press the tongue in the area of the cinguli of the lower central incisors (Fig. 1-17), and he is asked to pucker, grin, open wide and close. These facial gymnastics should be repeated three or four times.

10. After 5 minutes, remove the lower alginate impression using the air syringe (Fig. 1-18).

11. Follow step 11 for the pouring of upper impressions, pour and invert upwards (Fig. 1-19).

12. With both impressions completed, we proceed to the fabrication of custom-made acrylic trays.

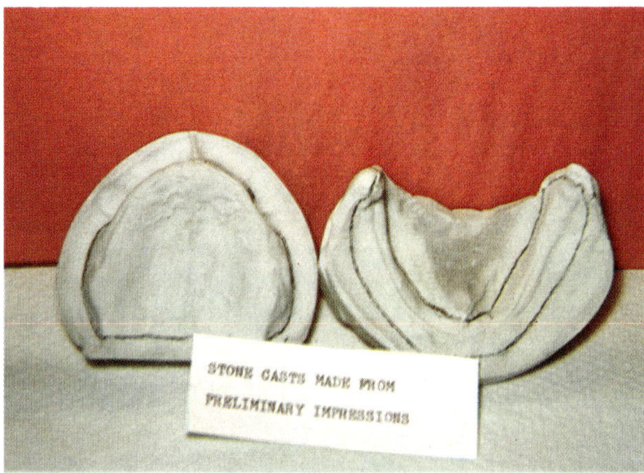

Fig. 2-1

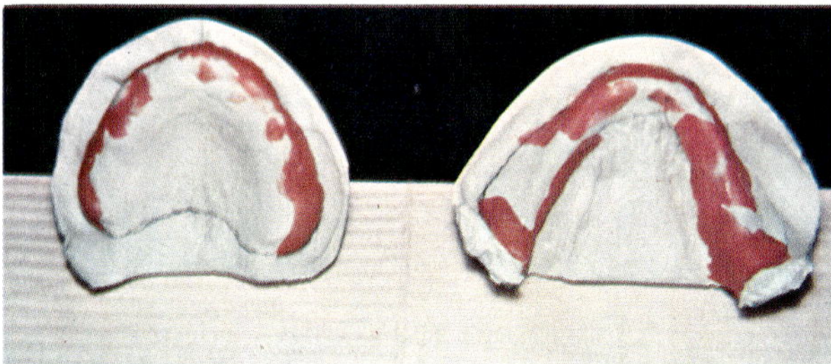

Fig. 2-2

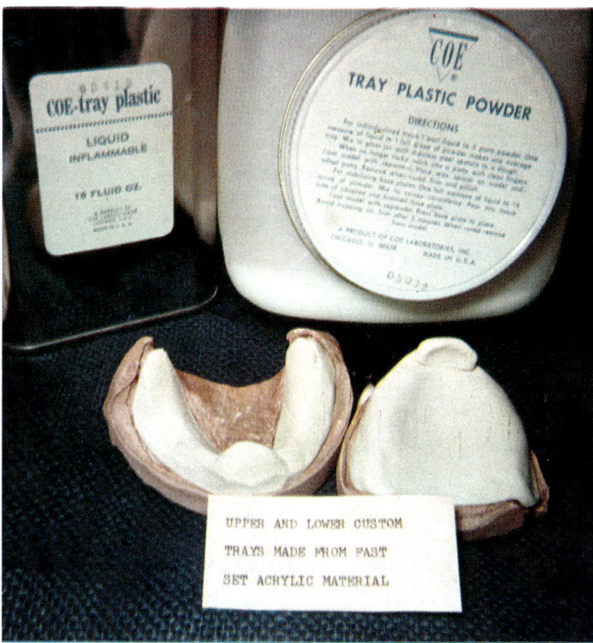

Fig. 2-3

2. Constructing Custom-made Acrylic Impression Trays

UPPER IMPRESSION TRAYS

1. Outline the preliminary stone casts with a soft pencil (Fig. 2-1) 2.0 mm. short of the mucobuccal fold, from the hamular notch on one side to the hamular notch on other.
2. Undercuts, if present, may be eliminated with soft wax (Fig. 2-2).
3. Make the upper impression tray using any fast tray acrylic. At this stage it is best to extend the tray posteriorly longer than necessary in order to ascertain the correct dimensions later when checking the length of the post-dam area.
4. Trim the tray to the outline of the cast. A hole may be made with a No. 12 round bur over the incisive foramen, which relieves the pressure when taking the wash impression.

LOWER IMPRESSION TRAYS

5. Outline the preliminary cast with a soft pencil 2 mm. short of the mucobuccal fold from the buccal side of the retromolar pad on one side to the same point on the opposite side, and, similarly, from the mucolingual fold of the retromolar area on one side to the same point on the opposite side (as was shown in step 1).
6. Eliminate undercuts with soft wax or plastercine.
7. Make the lower tray, using any fast-set tray acrylic.
8. Trim the tray to the outline of the cast.
9. We now have upper and lower custom-made acrylic trays (Fig. 2-3).

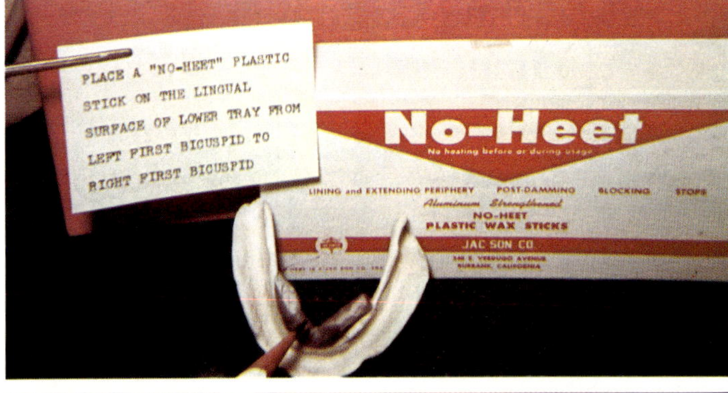

Fig. 3-1

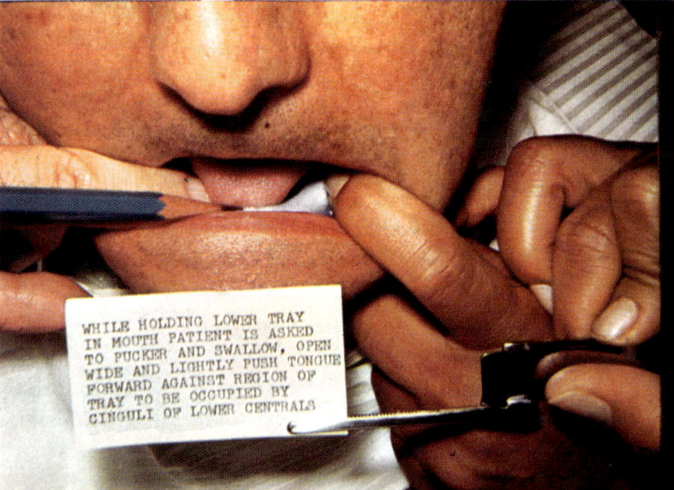

Fig. 3-2

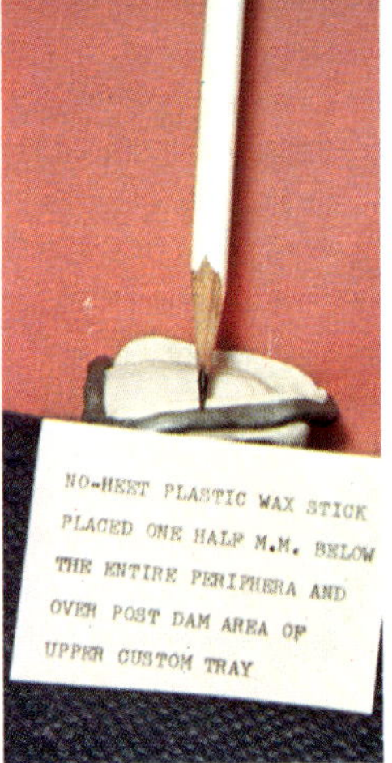

Fig. 3-3

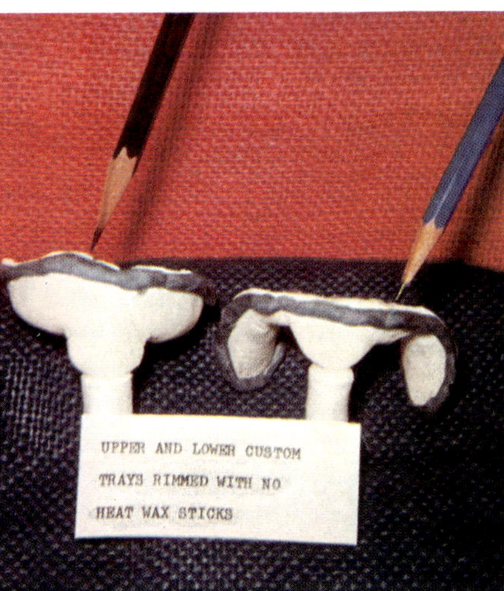

Fig. 3-4

3. Wash Impressions

1. Place a thick No-Heet* (Fig. 3-1) plastic wax stick on the lingual surface of the lower tray from the left first bicuspid to the right first bicuspid.
2. Place a thinned out No-Heet stick 0.5 mm. below the entire periphery of the lower tray from the lingual aspect of the first bicuspid on one side, joining the wax placed previously in the sublingual area, to the balance of the lingual flange—over the retromolar pads, around the buccal and labial aspects, over the retromolar pads to the lingual portion along the periphery, then joining the sublingual wax area on the other side.
3. Now place the lower rimmed-wax tray in the mouth. Ask the patient to extend his tongue slightly forward, gently pressing it into the region of the tray that corresponds to the cinguli of the lower central incisors (Fig. 3-2). Ask the patient to open his mouth wide, close and do mouth gymnastics in order to mold the No-Heet wax along the lower periphery.
4. Remove the lower tray from the mouth and proceed to the upper tray.
5. Rim the entire upper tray 0.5 to 1.0 mm. below the periphery with a thinned out No-Heet plastic wax stick (Fig. 3-3) from the buccal surface of one side, across the post-dam area, to the buccal surface of the opposite side.
   A. We now have upper and lower trays rimmed with wax stricks (Fig. 3-4).

*No-Heet Plastic Wax Sticks. Jac Son Co., 3416 West Victory Blvd., Burbank, Calif. 91505

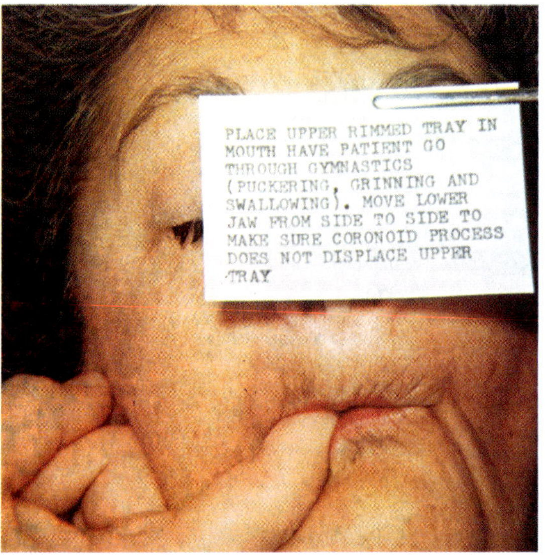

Fig. 3-5

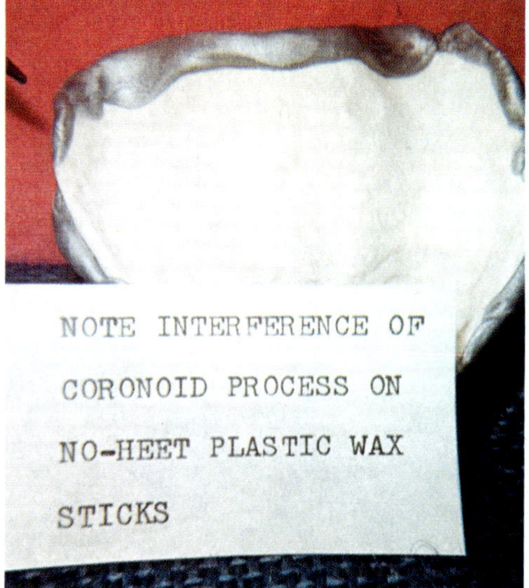

Fig. 3-6

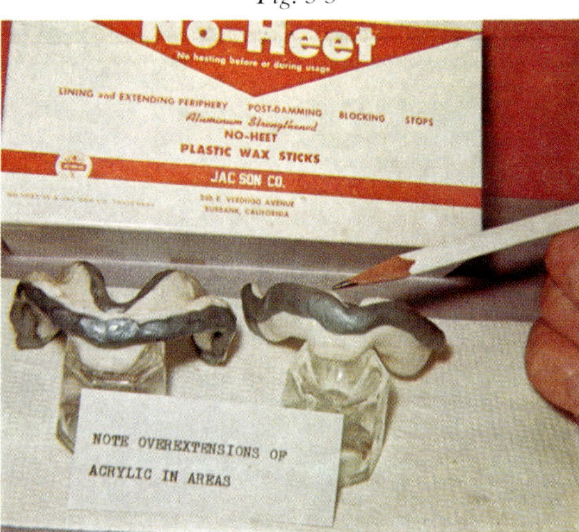

Fig. 3-7

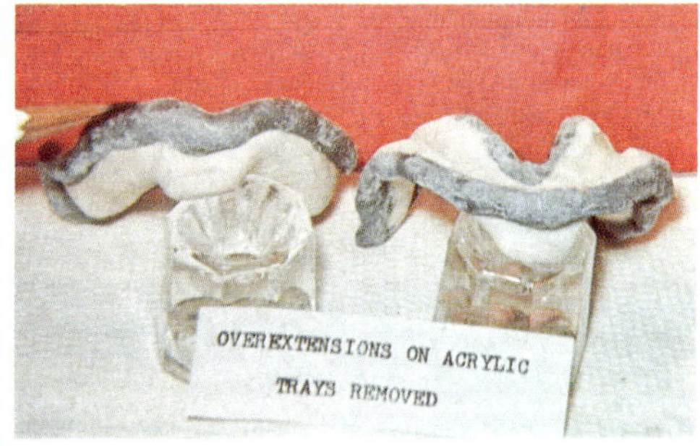

Fig. 3-8

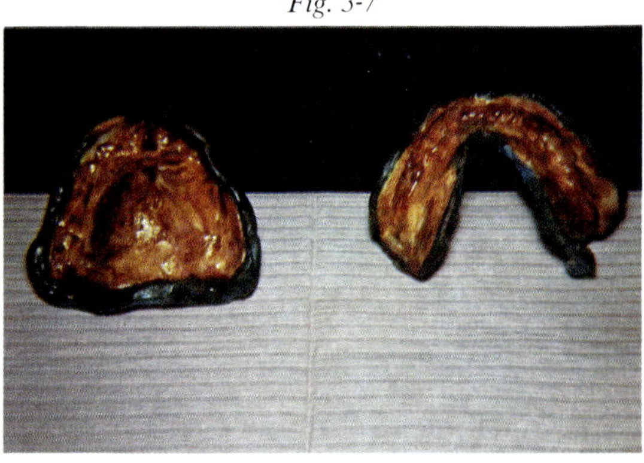

Fig. 3-9

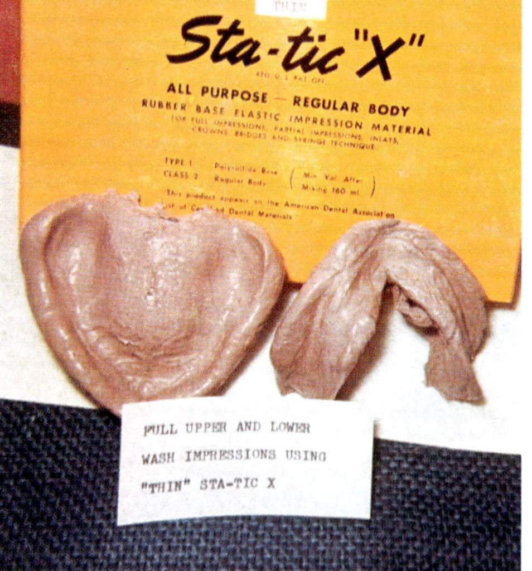

Fig. 3-10

6. Insert this upper wax-rimmed tray in the mouth and ask him to pucker, grin, suck, swallow and move the mandible from side to side (Fig. 3-5). This last step permits the proper lateral movement of the coronoid process of the mandible, and also provides for the preliminary border height and thickness of the buccal border of the upper denture that comes in contact in that region during the movement of the coronoid process. If this step is overlooked, the upper denture may become dislodged during function owing to interference (Fig. 3-6).

7. The upper tray is now removed from the mouth. Both the upper and lower wax-rimmed trays are examined for overextensions of acrylic along the periphery (Fig. 3-7).

8. By using sandpaper and a lathe, remove these acrylic overextensions (Fig. 3-8).

9. If you had not previously made the hole over the incisive foramen on the upper in order to relieve the pressure of the wash impression, make it now.

10. Apply Stalite* adhesive cement over that portion of the trays that is to receive rubber base material (Fig. 3-9).

11. In taking the lower impression, after mixing the material of choice according to the manufacturer's directions, load the tray with this material, have the patient rinse his mouth with a good astringent, and, after he has swallowed any excess saliva, ask him to open his mouth wide. The loaded tray is then introduced into the mouth. As soon as the tray is properly positioned, instruct him to close his mouth half way. Begin to seat the tray by first retracting with your fingers the buccal pouches of the cheeks so that they are not trapped in the impression. At the same time, as the tray is being seated (with a quivering motion), ask the patient to raise the tongue so that the lingual flabby tissues are not caught under the impression. As the tray is seated in place, instruct him to exert slight pressure with the tip of the tongue against the lingual area in which the cinguli of the lower anterior teeth will be placed. Now, while you are gently holding the lower tray down with the fingers of both hands, ask him to do mouth gymnastics, open wide and close, as was done when taking the preliminary alginate impression.

The patient is to continue mouth gymnastics for three minutes. Eight minutes after the loaded tray has been inserted, the material should have set. The lower impression then is removed from the mouth by either having the patient balloon out the cheeks or by using the air syringe around the periphery.

The upper wash impression is taken in a similar way, except that the tray is supported lightly with the index or second finger of one hand, and the patient is asked to pucker, grin and move the mandible from side to side to clear the coronoid process. These movements are continued for two or three minutes. After the material has set for eight minutes, the upper impression is removed from the mouth. We have now completed the upper and lower impressions (Fig. 3-10). For rubber base elastic impressions, I like to use Sta-tic X† or a special thin Sta-tic X material on a bad lower spinous ridge. These should be poured as soon as possible in a good stone composition. Boxing is not necessary.

---

*Sta-tic Elastic Cement. Stalite, Inc., Hialeah, Fla. 33013

†Sta-tic X Material by Stalite, Inc., 4480 East 11th Ave., Hialeah, Fla. 33013

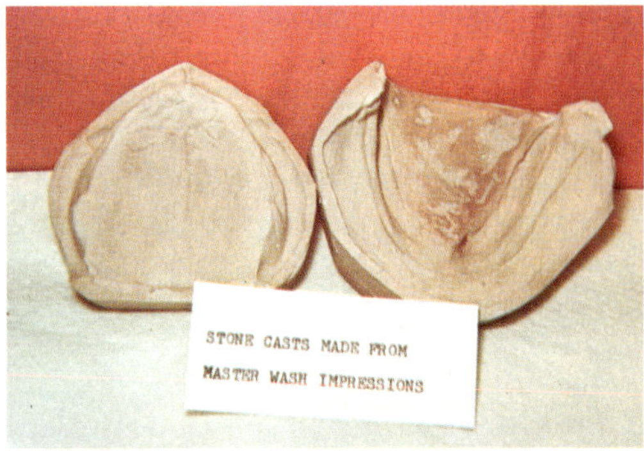

Fig. 4-1

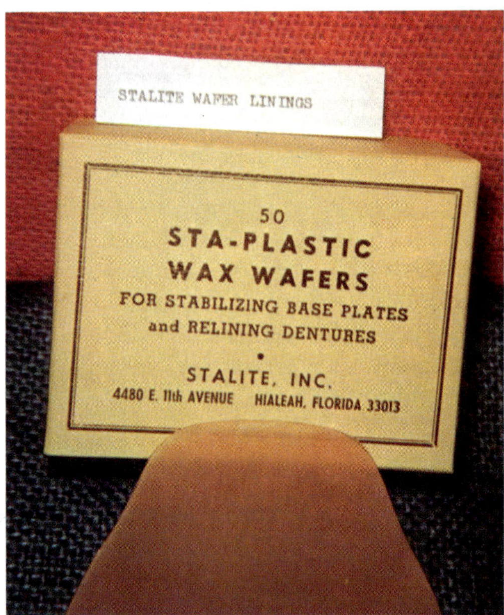

Fig. 4-2

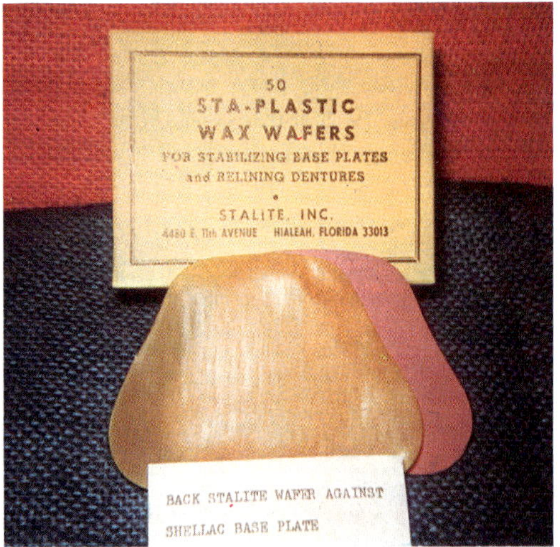

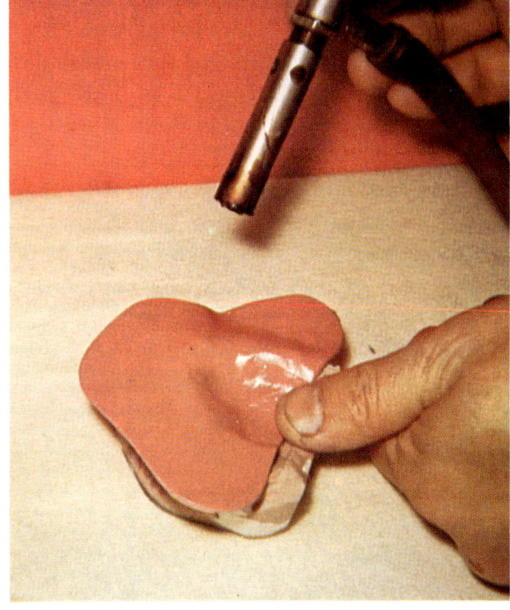

Fig. 4-4

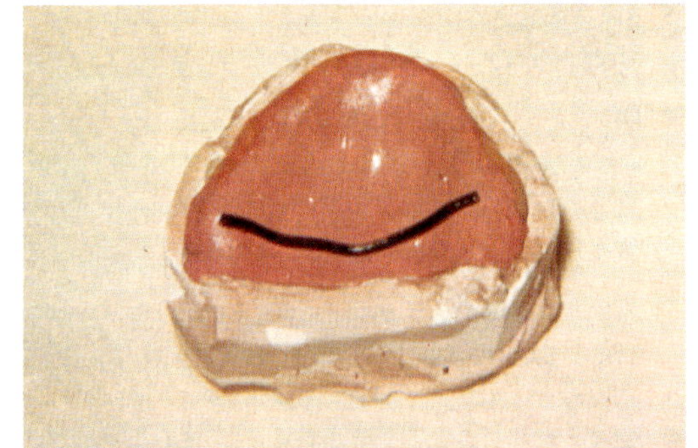

Fig. 4-5

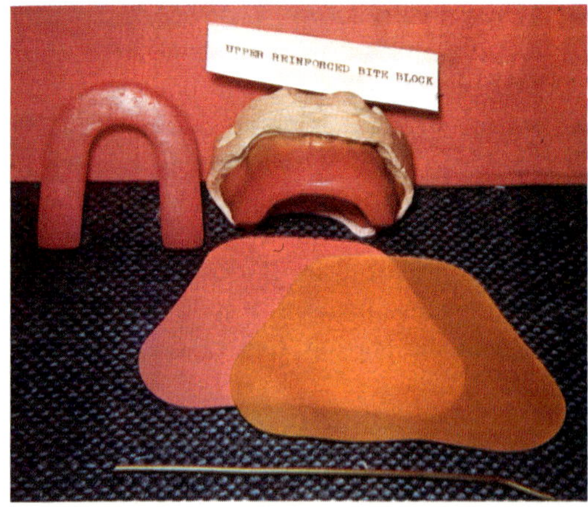

Fig. 4-6

Fig. 4-3

4. Building Bite Blocks From Wash Impressions

After the stone casts (Fig. 4-1) have been separated from the wash impressions, we proceed to build bite blocks on these casts. If shellac trays are reinforced by coat hanger wire and lined with plastic wafers* (Fig. 4-2), which facilitates removal from the models they are sturdy enough for the construction of wax rims and withstand the recording of centric and eccentric positions. The trays are built according to the following procedures.

UPPER BITE BLOCKS

1. Moisten the stone model in water.
2. Back a single-thickness base plate with a plastic wafer (Fig. 4-3).
3. Heat the base plate backed with the wafer over the stone cast until the mass drapes over it.
4. Adapt the mass to the cast with a moistened finger (Fig. 4-4).
5. Roll the edges of the mass around the periphery as far as the mucobuccal folds.
6. Insert the coat hanger wire across the post-dam area (Fig. 4-5), keeping it 4.0 to 5.0 mm. short of the posterior border in case shortening in this area is necessary when making adjustments for the length of the post-dam.
7. Trim off the excess boarders of the tray on a lathe, using sandpaper disks.
8. Place a hard-wax bite form† (Fig. 4-6) over the base plate and along the ridge from second molar to second molar.
9. Using a hot spatula, seal this wax rim to the tray.
10. Fill in the voids between the wax rim and the shellac tray by using a hard sheet wax.

---

*Sta-Plastic Wax Wafers. Stalite, Inc., 4480 E. 11th Ave., Hialeah, Fla. 33013

†Yates Rijform Bite Rims. Yates Mfg. Co., 1615 W. 15th St., Chicago, Ill. 60608 or Modern Materials Mfg. Co., St. Louis, Mo.

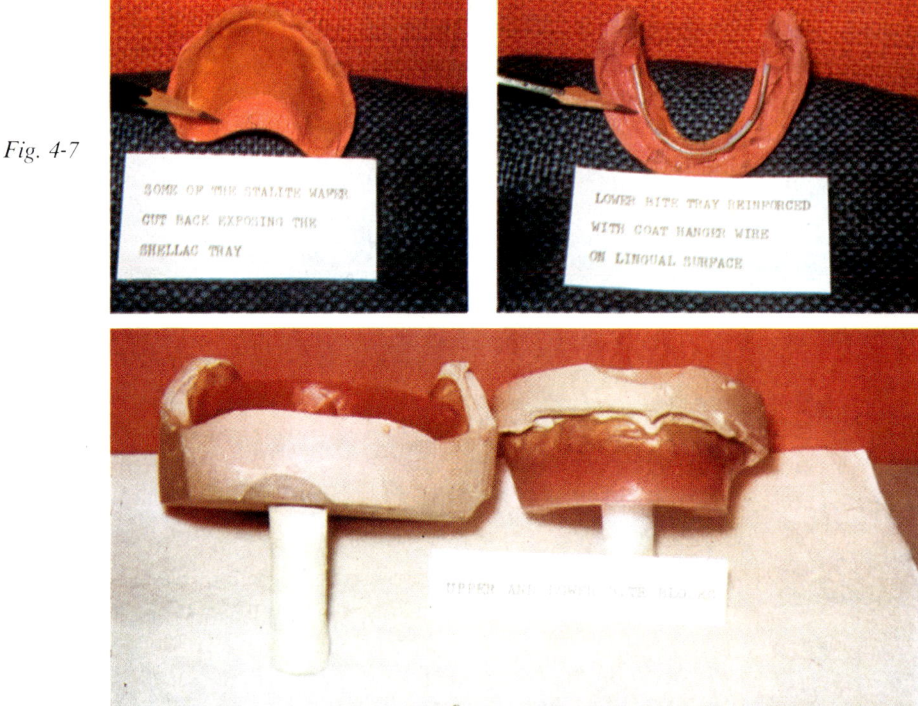

Fig. 4-7

Fig. 4-8

Fig. 4-9

11. Cut away some of the plastic wafer from the post-dam area (Fig. 4-7). This facilitates later checking in the post-dam area. We now have a finished maxillary bite block.

LOWER BITE BLOCKS

The procedure for the mandibular bite block is the same as that described for the maxillary bite block, with one exception—a very low rim of hard wax is placed on the tray so that soft wax can be superimposed at the time vertical and centric relation are recorded. The mandibular bite block should be reinforced with coat hanger wire on the lingual aspect (Fig. 4-8) from retromolar area to retromolar area.

The upper and lower bite blocks (Fig. 4-9) are now ready to be used for the recording of vertical and centric relation.

5. Preliminary Steps in Recording Vertical and Preliminary Centric Relation Through the Act of Swallowing

During the patient's first visit, when signs and symptoms were evaluated, we determined whether there was muscle spasm. If there was, we noted exactly where these areas of spasm existed. It is best to check these areas of possible spasm again, and inject each with a 2 per cent local anesthetic having no vasoconstrictor action. Remember, however, that it is not the local anesthetic per se that breaks the spasm, but the puncture of the needle. The small amount of local anesthetic prevents needle pain as we make several punctures in a one half inch circle in the area of the spasm. Why must we be concerned about muscle spasm? Because before we can record *correct* vertical and centric relation, and be able to repeat the same recording, it is essential to eliminate muscle spasms. The muscles most frequently involved are the external and internal pterygoids, although the masseters, temporals and a few lesser muscles of deglutition may be involved also.

THE DENTAL CHAIR

A dental chair must be so designed that the patient's head, neck, arms and legs feel absolutely relaxed. This relaxation factor alone is worth a good deal to me, especially when I am recording vertical and centric occlusion. In my opinion, the Virginia Chair meets these requirements better than other makes of chairs I have used in the past.

TECHNIC OF BREAKING MUSCLE SPASM

1. After checking the attachments of the internal pterygoid muscle with the left hand (Fig. 5-1), in the same region and in the same manner as one would palpate for a mandibular injection, apply light pressure medially just above the lingual bony prominence. Observe whether the patient exhibits pain. (If a spasm is present it is usually unnecessary to ask the patient whether he feels pain: just watching him wince is enough.) In checking for spasm in the internal pterygoid region, one must remember to avoid any sharp lingula, so as to avoid a false response to the pressure applied.

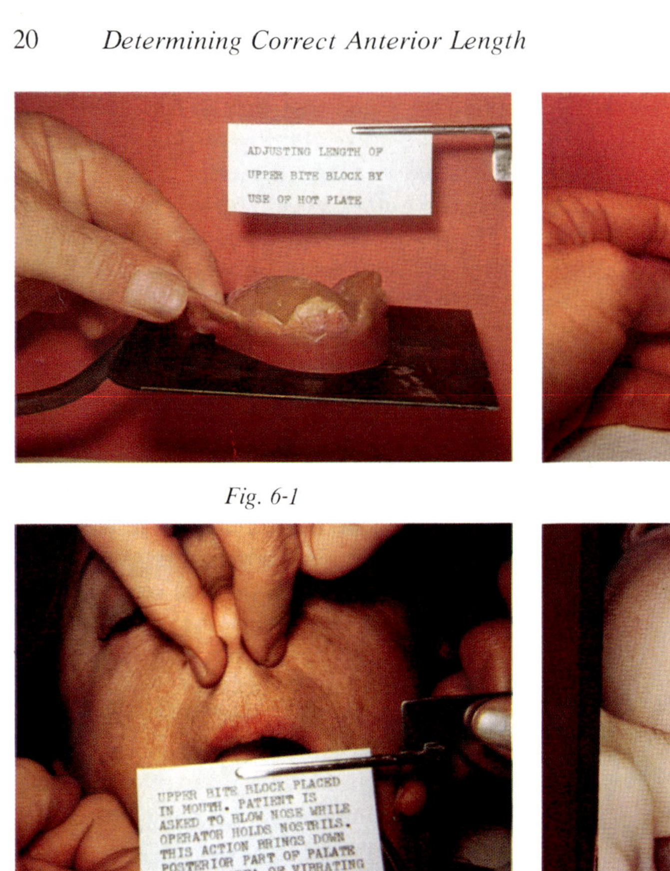

Fig. 6-1

Fig. 6-2

Fig. 6-3

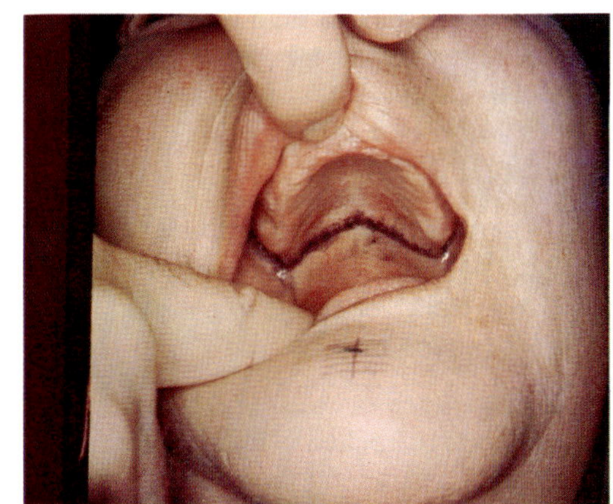

Fig. 6-4

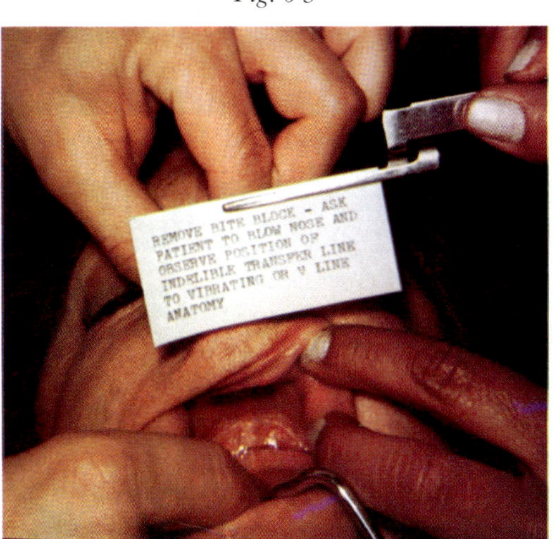

Fig. 6-5

Fig. 6-6

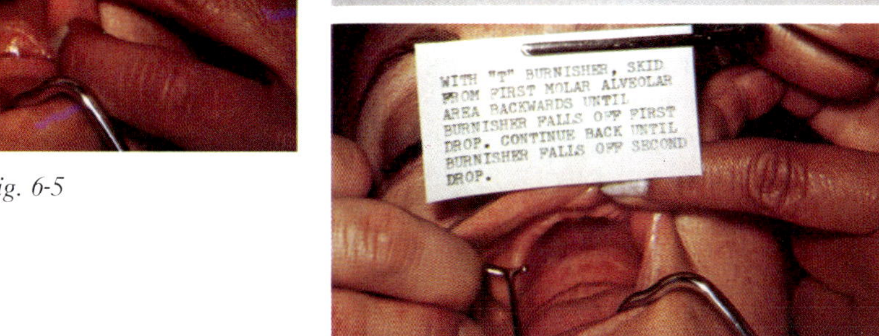

Fig. 6-7

6. Determining Correct Anterior Length; Placement of the Post-dam in the Upper Bite Block

When all the muscle spasms have been relieved, you are ready to record vertical and centric relation. First, establish the correct occlusal height by the use of a hot plate to reduce wax length (Fig. 6-1). Then establish the correct anterior length of the bite block and the placement of the post-dam. This is accomplished in the following manner:

OCCLUSAL HEIGHT

If the patient who comes to us is already edentulous, photographs showing the former profile of his natural teeth are a great aid in determining the length of the upper anterior bite block. However, if there are no pre-extraction photographs or records showing the extent to which the patient displayed his natural teeth, we are forced to determine the length of the upper bite block by other means.

One guide to determine how much of the teeth to show is the age of the patient—the older the patient, the less teeth we will show (and the shorter the bite block); the younger the patient, the more teeth we will show (and the longer the bite block).

PLACEMENT OF THE POST-DAM

The post-dam area should always be established by the dentist and not by the dental technician. I do not believe in using the foramen palatinae as a means of determining the length of the denture because the foramen palatinae are sometimes anterior, and sometimes posterior, to the point at which the denture should end. Therefore, if you ask your technician always to build the posterior portion of the bite block a little longer than necessary, you can establish the correct length yourself. This is done in the following manner:

1. With an indelible pencil, mark well the entire distal end of the bite block (Fig. 6-2) on the palatal side from tuberosity to tuberosity, that portion that will come in contact with the palate when placed in the mouth.
2. Using a cotton roll, dry the patient's palate.
3. Insert the marked bite block into the patient's mouth.
4. While holding the patient's nose with two fingers of one hand, and while holding down the tongue with one or two fingers of your other hand, in order to avoid the tongue obliterating the marking, have him blow his nose (Fig. 6-3). This causes the palate to descend and contact the pencil marking on the bite block, leaving a tracing of this mark across its distal portion.
5. Remove the bite block from the mouth while still holding down the tongue, and observe the transmitted line across the post-dam area (Fig. 6-4).
6. Place two fingers on his nose and ask him to blow his nose again.

   Observe how the marked distal portion of the palate descends in relationship to the "V" formed at the break of the hard and soft palate (Fig. 6-5). This break—or descent at an angle of the soft palate—is also referred to as the vibrating line.

7. If your original marking was too long (too far toward the throat and therefore away from the vibrating line), cut the

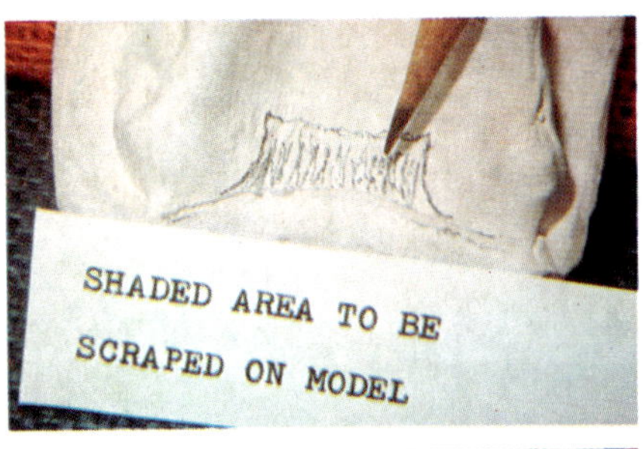

Fig. 6-8

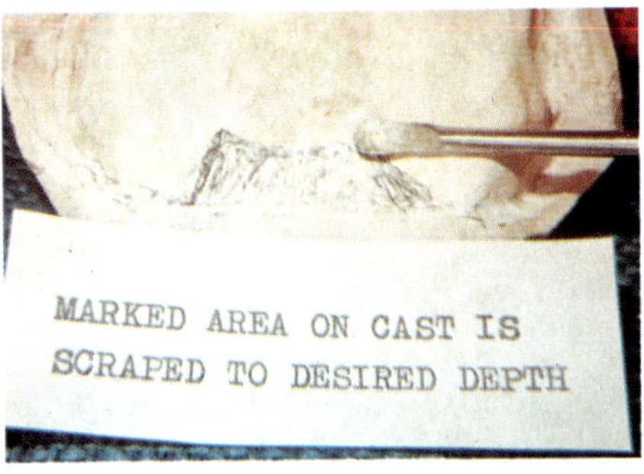

Fig. 6-9

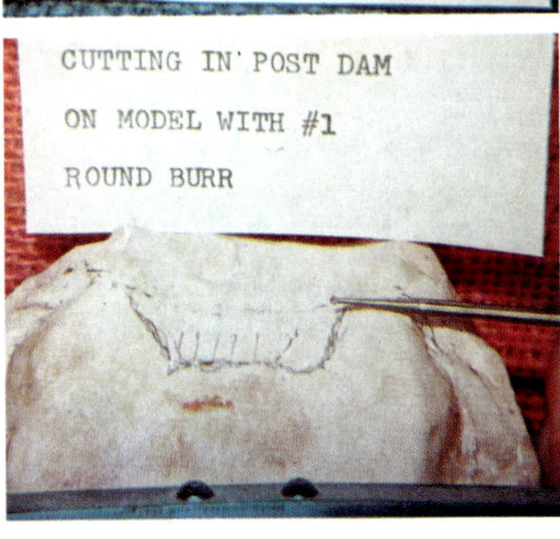

Fig. 6-10

bite block back from the vibrating line toward the throat until it is 1.5 to 2.0 mm. past the vibrating line.

8. If the bite block is anterior to the vibrating line, extend it until it is about 1.5 to 2.0 mm. past the vibrating line.

9. Transfer the corrections in length made by the bite block to the model (Fig. 6-6), and with a No. 1 round bur, cut in on the cast, about one millimeter depth, the distal aspect of the bite block from tuberosity to tuberosity.

10. Now, to locate the area over the hamular notch, the following procedure is employed: Start skidding a "T" burnisher (Fig. 6-7) from the molar ridge area back toward the throat. As you keep going back you literally "fall off a cliff"; as you continue to skid back, you will feel another drop-off. End the denture bite block at the second drop-off.

11. Make a notation of this point on your stone model.

12. Palpate with a ball burnisher the amount of movable tissue present in the mouth between the two hamular notches and, with a pencil, roughly transfer this outline to the cast (Fig. 6-8) by shading the model. This indicates approximately the amount the cast may be scraped (Fig. 6-9) in the post-dam area to create a better seal between the hard and soft areas of the palate. At the distal end following the pencil mark on the cast, cut in with a No. 1 round bur (Fig. 6-10) about one mm. in depth depending on the compressibility of the tissues. The scraping gradually lessens as we come forward anteriorly. As we scrape the cast we try to follow the anatomy of the hard palate at that point.

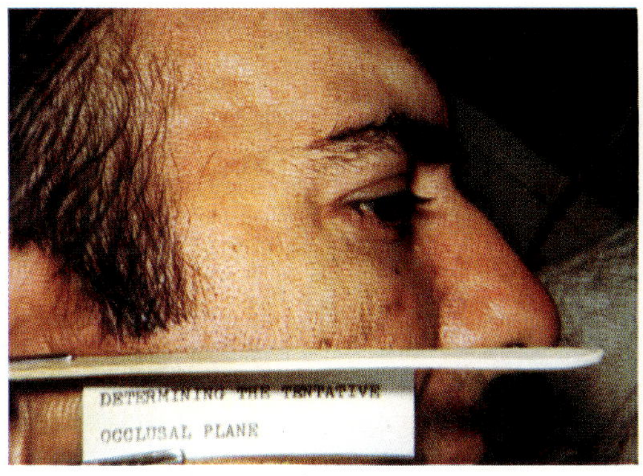

Fig. 7-1

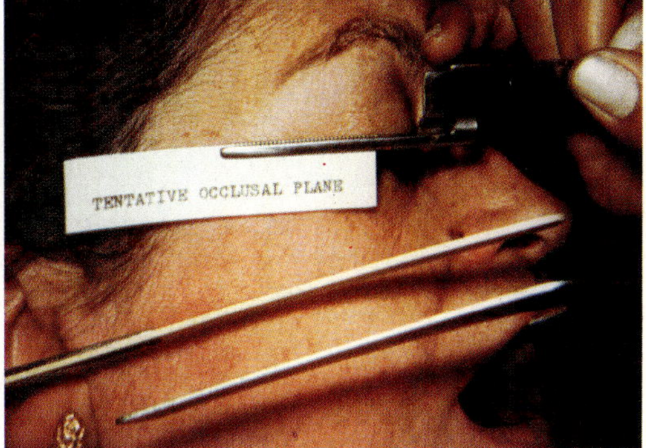

Fig. 7-2

7. Determining the Occlusal Plane

The occlusal plane, as defined in a glossary of prosthodontic terms, is an imaginary surface which is related anatomically to the cranium and which theoretically touches the incisal edges of the incisors and tips of the occluding surfaces of the posterior teeth. It is not a plane in the true sense of the word but represents the mean of the curvature of the surface.

It is the author's experience that the determination of the occlusal plane in a problem case is very important. This phase is thoroughly described in Chapter 12 of my book, *An Atlas of Complete Denture Prosthesis.* In that chapter, I describe how to avoid an unfavorable occlusal plane so that the patient experiences no difficulty in removing food from the denture table and dislodging the lower denture, or in biting the lateral borders of the tongue. Since here I am describing non-problem cases, I shall simplify the procedure.

After establishing the anterior length on the bite block, a workable arbitrary occlusal plane is established in the following manner:

Using the fixed points of the tragus of the ear (Fig. 7-1) and the ala of the nose as landmarks, we try by means of tongue depressors or a Fox gauge to establish a line from the posterior to the anterior of the bite block as parallel as possible to the tragus-ala line. Many times it will be necessary to shave off the wax on the posterior occlusal surfaces of the bite block until we achieve a state of parallelism (Fig. 7-2) between the tragus-ala line and the bite block.

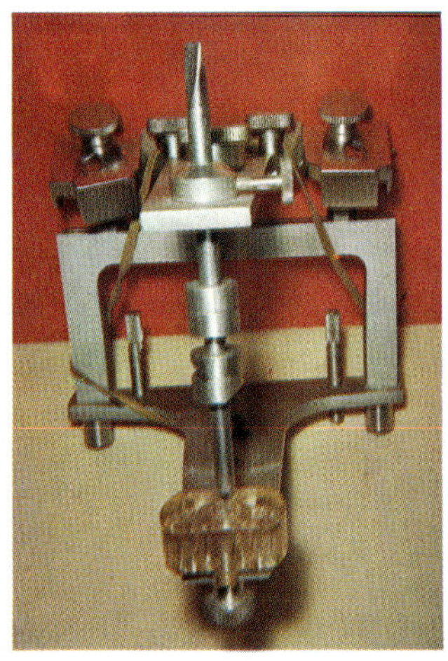

Fig. 8-1

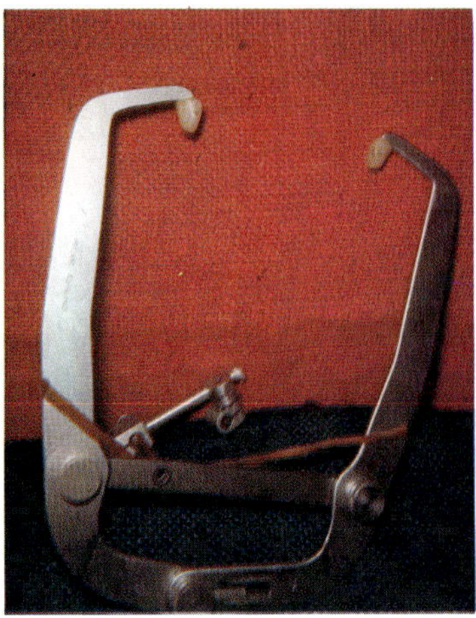

Fig. 8-2

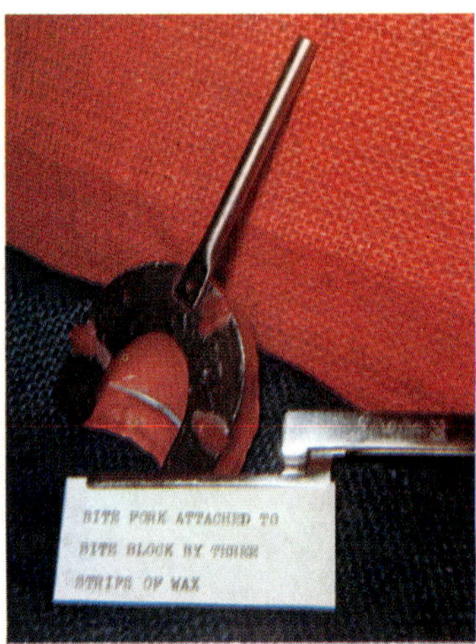

Fig. 8-3

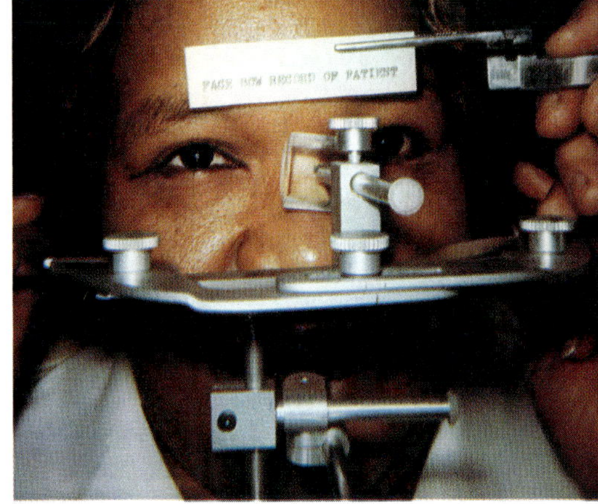

Fig. 8-4

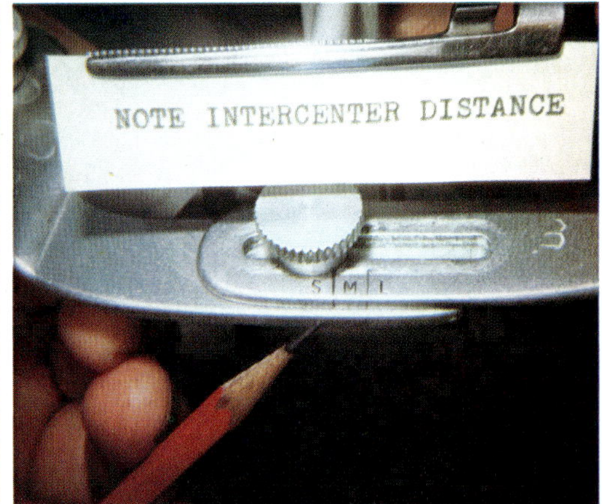

Fig. 8-5

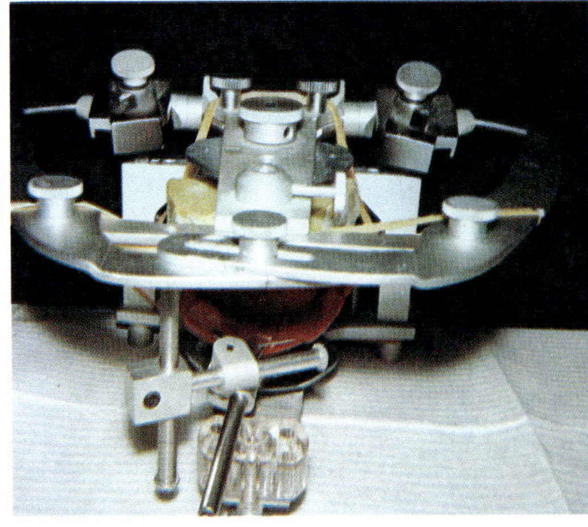

Fig. 8-6

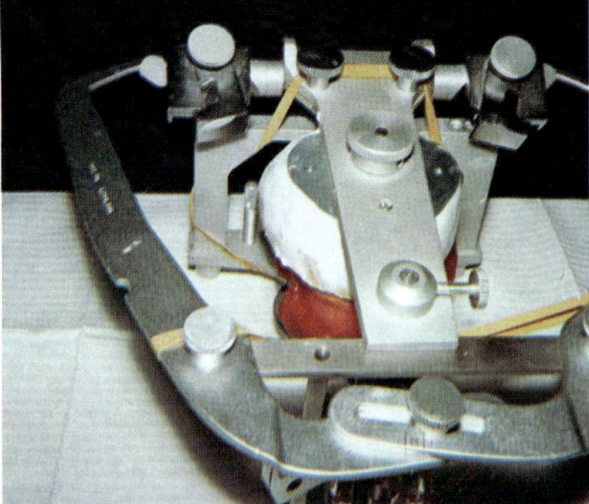

Fig. 8-7

8. The Face Bow Recording

There are many articulators on the market that can be used in the construction of dentures; however, since the Whip-Mix* articulator (Fig. 8-1) is a simple to use, semi-adjustable instrument, I find that for non-problem denture cases it is an excellent instrument upon which to construct dentures. Therefore, employing the Whip-Mix articulator, our next step is to take a face bow recording.

1. Attach the Whip-Mix face bow (Fig. 8-2) to the upper bite block (Fig. 8-3) by locking it in securely with wax in three or four areas.

2. Place this bite block, with the bite fork attached, in the mouth and, following the excellent instruction bulletin that comes with the Whip-Mix articulator, slip the "ice tongue" face bow over and into the handle of the bite fork. Make sure that the patient guides the ear pieces of the face bow into the external auditory meatuses. At this time position and center the plastic nose piece (the third point of reference) on the nose and tighten all the screws. The face bow record is now tightly secured on the head of the patient (Fig. 8-4). At this time notice the intercondylar, or, as preferred by some, the intercenter distance (Fig. 8-5). This is marked "S" for small, "M" for medium and "L" for large.

3. Remove the third point of reference from the assembly and remove the entire face bow record (attached face bow and bite block) from the mouth.

4. Following the instructions either in the Whip-Mix booklet or in my Atlas, mount this face bow record on the articulator (Fig. 8-6) and slide the upper cast into place on the bite block.

5. Articulate the upper cast to the articulator by means of a good plaster composition (Fig. 8-7).

6. When the stone has set, remove the face bow apparatus from the articulator; also remove the upper bite block from the articulator. This bite block is now to be used in the recording of vertical and preliminary centric relation through the act of swallowing. When vertical and preliminary centric relation are recorded, we will return to this in order to complete our articulation on the instrument.

*Whip-Mix Corp., Louisville, Ky.

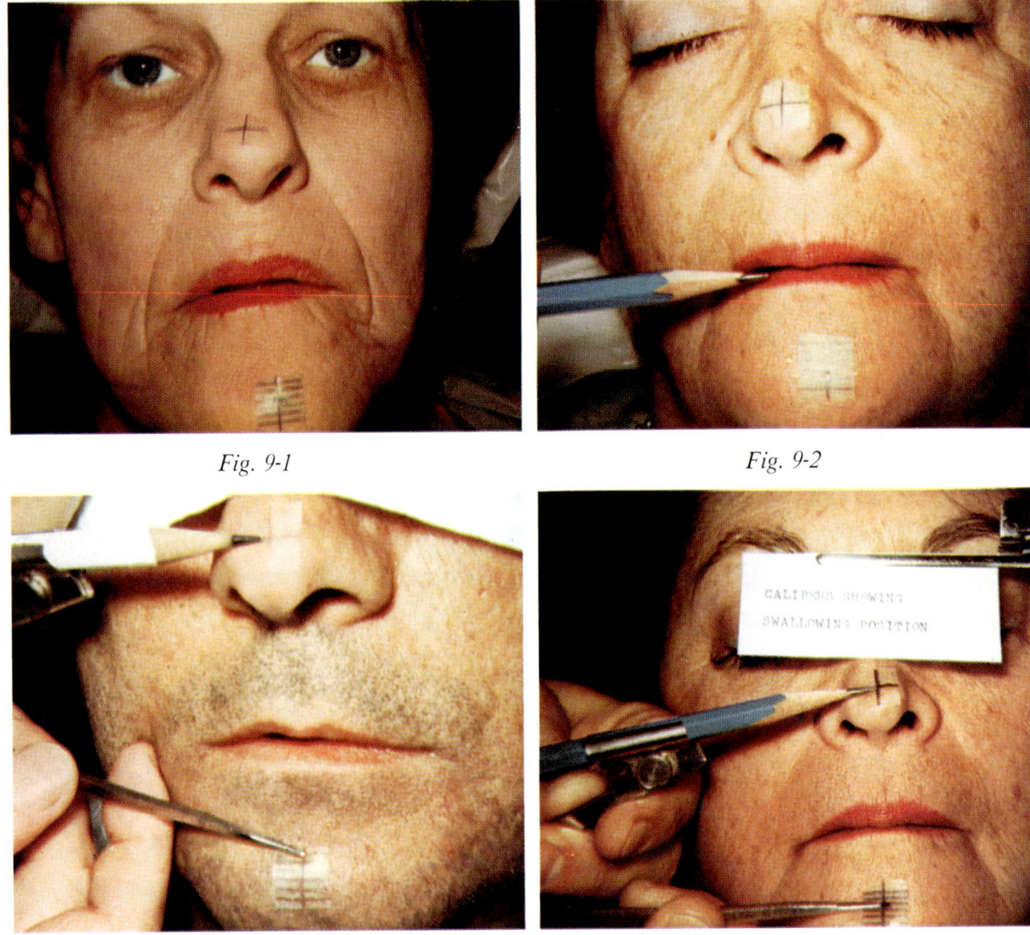

Fig. 9-1

Fig. 9-2

Fig. 9-3

Fig. 9-4

9. Recording Vertical and Preliminary Centric Relation Through the Act of Swallowing

1. Place one piece of tape marked with "+" on the tip of the patient's nose and a second marked with a vertical line intersected by 4 or 5 horizontal lines (spaced about 2.0 mm. apart), on his chin (Fig. 9-1).

   Making sure that the spasms are still completely absent, we can proceed with the recording of vertical and preliminary centric relation through the act of swallowing.

2. We place in the mouth the same maxillary bite block that was used in the face bow recording, adjusted to the correct lip line, correct post-dam length and to the tragus-ala occlusal plane.

3. Ask the patient to sit erect and to lick his lips while repeating the word "Emma." He should relax, and should ignore your movements while you take measurements.

4. When you know that the patient is relaxed, and after he has said the word "Emma" three or four times, his lips should be slightly apart (Fig. 9-2). At this juncture measure with calipers the distance between the "+" on the nose and the upper most horizontal line on the chin (Fig. 9-3). This distance indicates the "rest position" of the mandible. Actually, the rest position when teeth are present is revealed by the distance or space between the teeth when the jaws are apart.

5. Once you have determined the rest position (which should be verified by repeating the measurement several times), determine the free-way space.
   A. While holding one end of the calipers on the nose mark "+" and the other end slightly away from (not touching) the chin markings (1/8 in. is adequate clearance), ask the patient to swallow.
   B. Observe at the "peak" of the swallow which horizontal mark on the chin is aligned with the end of the calipers (Fig. 9-4). (Because at this time there is no lower bite block in the mouth, the patient swallows upward, toward the nose mark, without interference.)
   C. By counting the horizontal marks crossed during the act of swallowing, you can determine easily how many millimeters of free-way space the patient needs. An old fashioned but unfortunately still popular belief is that a 3.0 mm. free-way space is universally adequate.

      I have observed patient's exhibiting adequate free-way space of 5.0, 7.0, 9.0, 11.0 and 13.0 mm. Furthermore, it has been my experience that if an individually inadequate free-way space is not recognized and provided, the case will fail. If we do not allow for an adequate space, nature will attempt to provide one at the expense of underlying structures.

We must measure free-way space accurately and not rely only upon appearance and approximations. The fact that the upper and lower bite blocks make the face look well and fill out the mouth does not imply necessarily that the free-way space is adequate. It is well known that an open or a closed vertical, especially the former, causes temporomandibular joint symptoms and the problems that go with them.

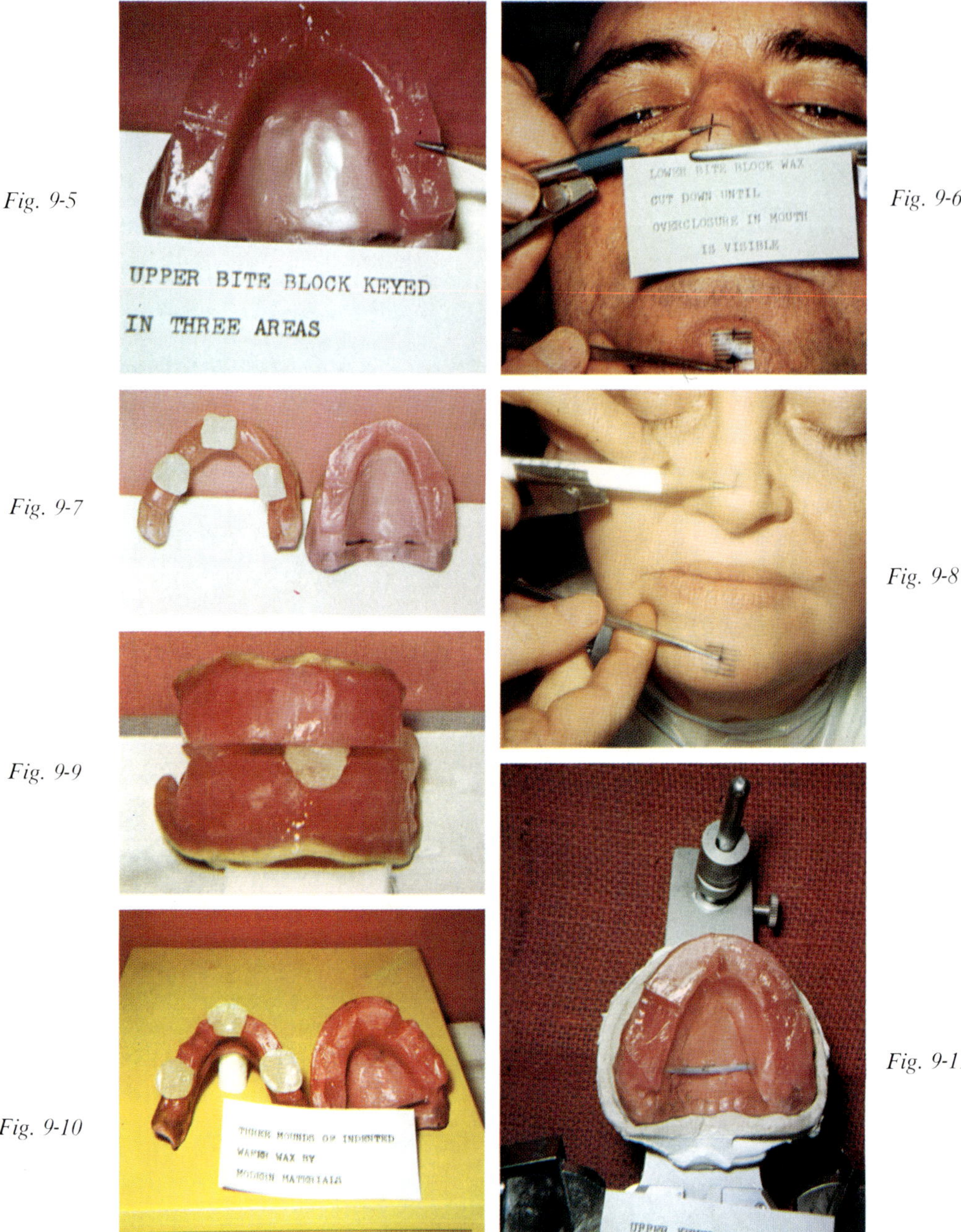

Fig. 9-5

Fig. 9-6

Fig. 9-7

Fig. 9-8

Fig. 9-9

Fig. 9-10

Fig. 9-11

I recommend that the measurement described here for determining the correct free-way space be repeated several times to insure accuracy. After some practice you will be gratified to find that you are able to record this free-way space over and over again, obtaining the same results each time.

To recapitulate, what does measurement of the range of motion during swallowing really mean? Simply that the lower most horizontal line reached by the caliper during the swallow reveals the patient's jaw closure when, with the lower bite block in the mouth, he contacts the upper bite block. In other words, it is in this position and at this point that the patient's upper and lower teeth contact during the last stage of deglutition. When his jaws open and he assumes the rest position again, the distance between the jaws constitutes the free-way space. Thus the free-way space is the amount of space that should be present between the jaws when they are apart in physiologic rest.

6. Once you have recorded with calipers the rest position on the chin, key the upper bite block in the right and left molar and anterior regions (Fig. 9-5), applying ample petrolatum to all three regions.

7. Now replace the upper bite block in the mouth. Insert the lower bite block in the mouth also, and ask the patient to bring the upper and lower jaws together. Measure with the calipers to see if wax—and how much wax— has to be removed from the lower in order to arrive at a definite overclosure of the vertical according to the nose-chin markings (Fig. 9-6).

8. Leaving the upper bite block in the mouth, remove the lower bite block and place upon it 3 mounds of soft wax* (Fig. 9-7) opposite the keys of the upper bite block.

9. Heat the wax mounds slightly with an alcohol torch.

10. Lightly powder the upper and lower bite blocks with a good adhesive.

11. Insert the lower bite block in the patient's mouth, and, using either a mint candy on the tongue (as described in my book in steps 11 and 12, page forty-nine) or—a quicker and better method—asking the patient to relax the lower jaw, with your right hand gently guide the mandible back to the most terminal position possible. Ask the patient to begin closing the jaws together in this position until you see that slight contact is being made on the 3 mounds of soft wax. Now ask him to bring the upper and lower lips together. Remove your hand from the chin and ask him to swallow, holding that position. While the patient is holding this swallow position, ask him to swallow every 20 or 30 seconds about 3 or 4 times until your established occlusal vertical dimension has been reached (Fig. 9-8).

    Remember that as long as we do not tell the patient to bite, he will not overswallow, provided of course that the pterygoid muscles are not in spasm.

12. With ice water thoroughly chill both upper and lower bite blocks while still in the mouth.

13. Remove the bite blocks from the mouth intact (Fig. 9-9).

14. Separate the upper bite block from the lower, whose wax attachments are indented (Fig. 9-10).

15. Place the upper keyed bite block back on the previously mounted cast on the articulator (Fig. 9-11).

*Wafer Wax, Modern Materials.

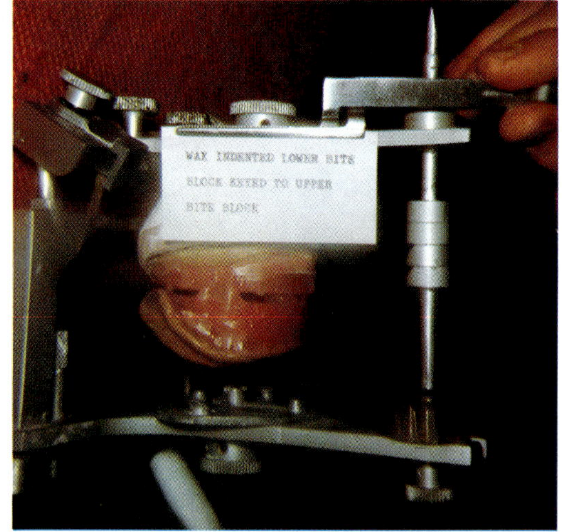

Fig. 9-12

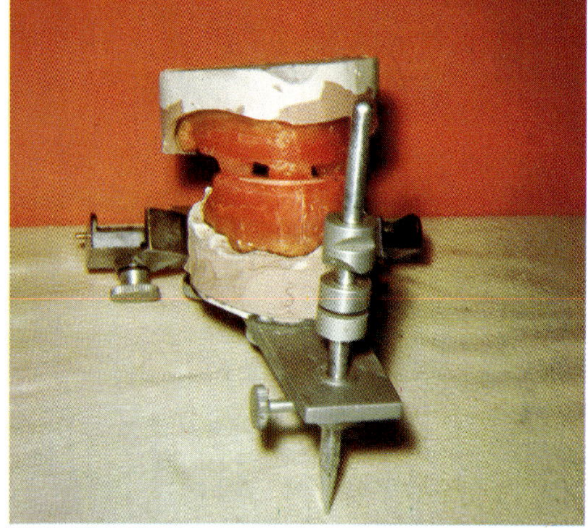

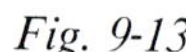
Fig. 9-13

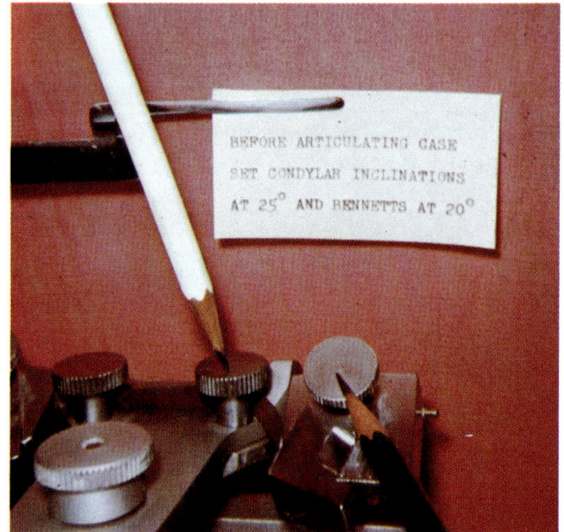

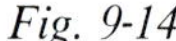
Fig. 9-14

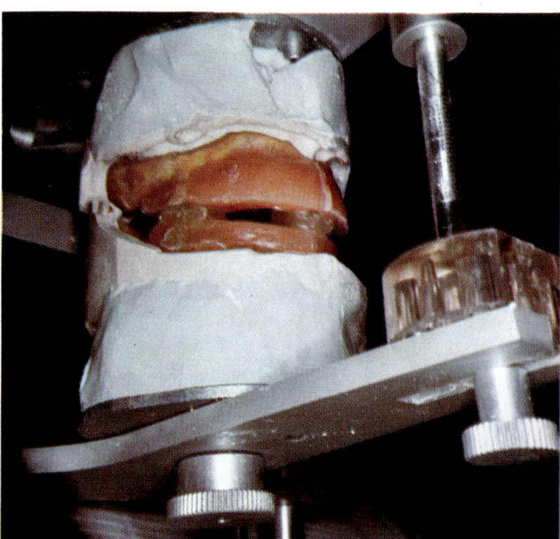

Fig. 9-15

16. Fit the wax-indented lower bite block to the keyed upper bite block (Fig. 9-12).

17. Insert the lower cast into the lower bite block (Fig. 9-13).
    A. Before finishing the articulation, set the condylar inclinations at 25 degrees or 30 degrees and the Bennetts at 20 degrees (Fig. 9-14).

18. Finish the articulation (Fig. 9-15).

At this stage, if you wish to recheck centric occlusion, remove the indented soft wax on the lower and replace the 3 mounds with new soft wax. Remove the bite blocks from the articulator and replace them in the mouth. Then recheck these re-swallowed-in bite blocks on the articulator. Your recordings will be the same if the steps were followed exactly.

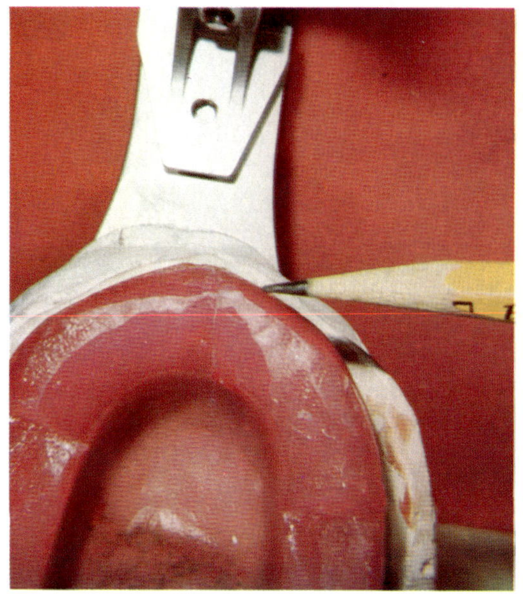

Fig. 10-1

Fig. 10-2

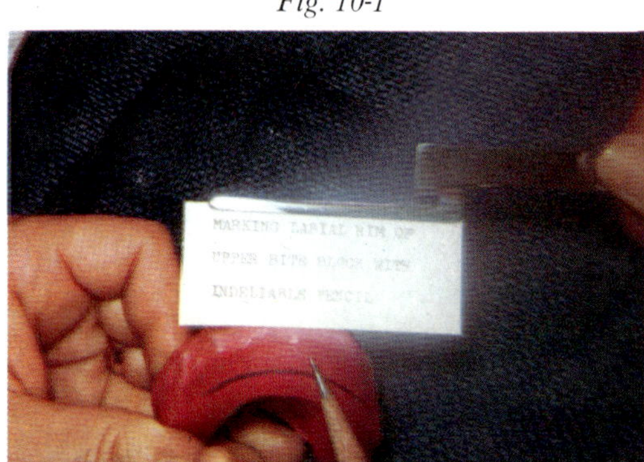

Fig. 10-3

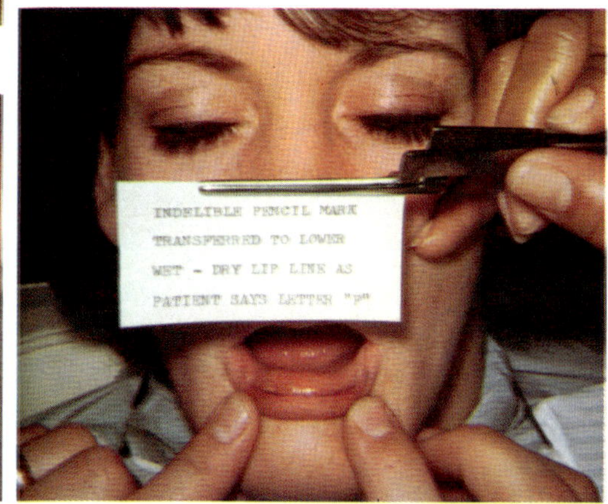

Fig. 10-4

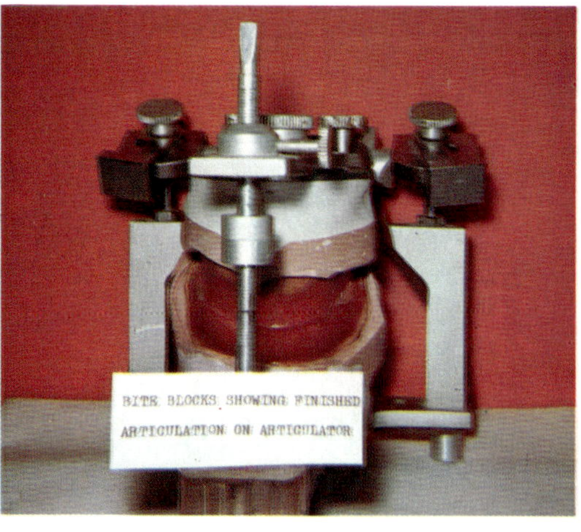

Fig. 10-5

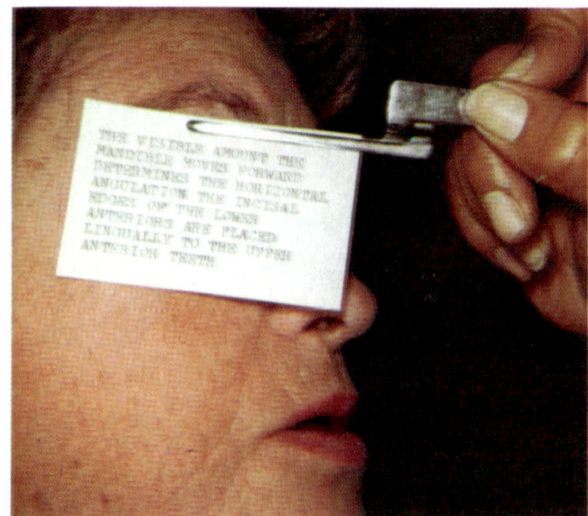

Fig. 10-6

10. The Positioning of the Anterior Teeth

THE "F" SOUND AND THE SETTING OF THE MAXILLARY ANTERIOR TEETH*

During the establishment of the occlusal plane we determined approximately the anterior lip length of the maxillary bite block. Now the anterior section of this wax bite block can be shaped from cuspid to cuspid (Fig. 10-1), and this should be done in such a way as to conform to the wet-dry line of the lower lip when the patient slowly repeats the letter "F" (Fig. 10-2). In other words, keep cutting or adding wax to this segment of the bite block until the wax lightly contacts and seals the wet-dry line on the lower lip from cuspid to cuspid. Check this position of seal by marking the labial portion of maxillary bite block with an indelible pencil (Fig. 10-3), and then have him say the word "F" again until this line is transferred to the dry-wet line of lower (Fig. 10-4). If sufficient time is spent it is possible to contour the maxillary bite block so that the teeth can be positioned correctly from this contour. Nonetheless, when checking esthetics and phonetics, it may be necessary to make slight alterations in the positioning of the maxillary teeth so placed.

THE "S" SOUND AND THE SETTING OF THE MANDIBULAR ANTERIOR TEETH*

After the maxillary anterior wax bite block has been adjusted, we turn our attention to the anterior section of the mandibular bite block in order to determine how far lingually or labially to set the mandibular anterior teeth.

One way to determine this is to follow the procedure described on pages 54 and 55 in my book *An Atlas of Complete Dentures*. Alternatively, remove both bite blocks from the articulator, insert these bite blocks into the mouth, and ask the patient to gently retrude the lower jaw to centric position. Make sure that the wax on the upper bite block is flush with the wax on the lower, as was the case when they were first removed from the articulator (Fig. 10-5).

1. Ask the patient to count from 60 to 70 several times. As he pronounces the sound "S" during the count, observe how far the mandible moves forward (Fig. 10-6), if it moves at all. The more the mandible moves forward the more overjet will be needed. In other words, the mandibular anterior teeth will be placed farther lingually in relation to the lingual surfaces of the maxillary anteriors. Adjust the lower softened wax to this position on the bite block by either bending this labial wax lingually or by removing more of the wax on the labial portion.

   The final test for phonetics and esthetics during the try-in usually determines the amount of overbite. However, in the case of the trial set-up for the upper and lower anteriors, a good rule is to introduce about the same degree of vertical overlap as was necessary in the horizontal overbite. The amount of overbite and overjet is usually referred to as "incisal guidance."

---

*Pound, E.: *Esthetics and phonetics*. J. Prosthet. Dent. Oct., 1966.

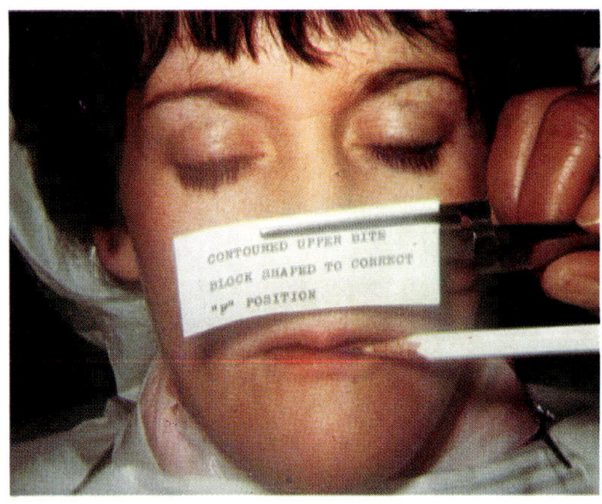

Fig. 11-1

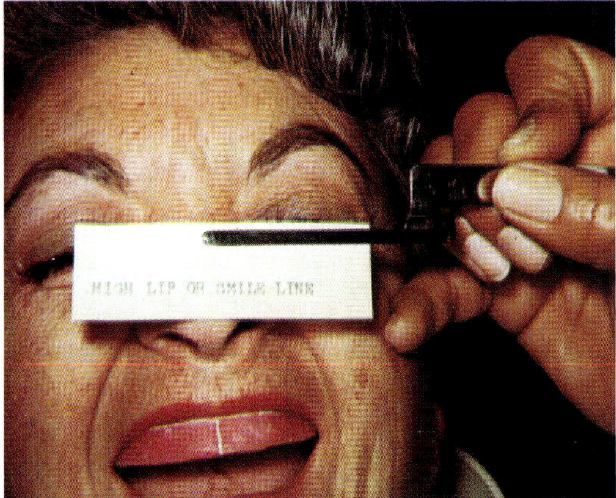

Fig. 11-2

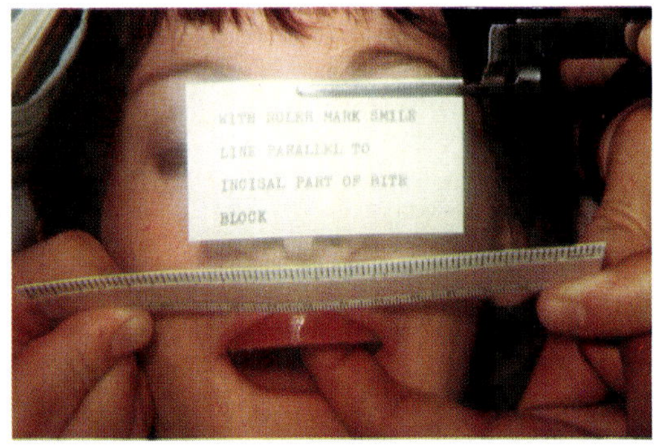

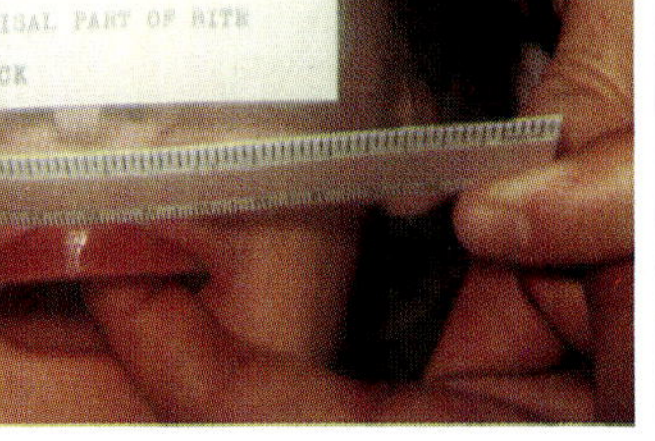

Fig. 11-3

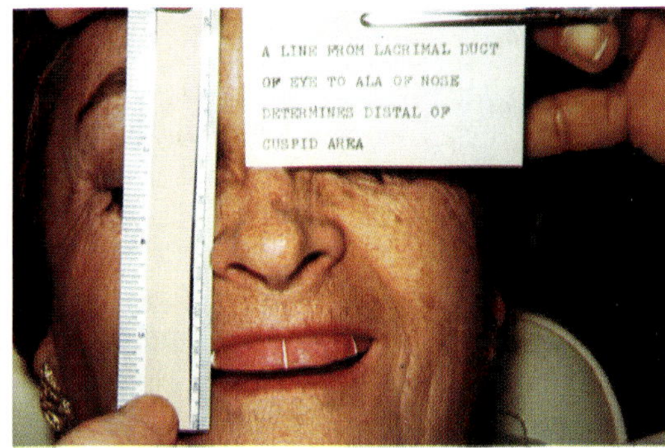

Fig. 11-4

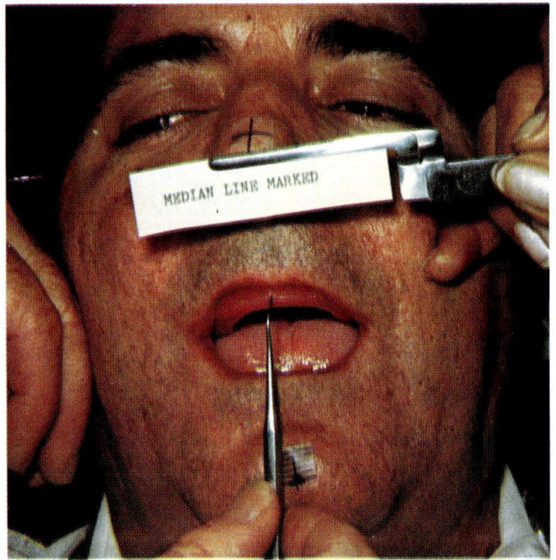

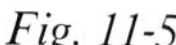

Fig. 11-5

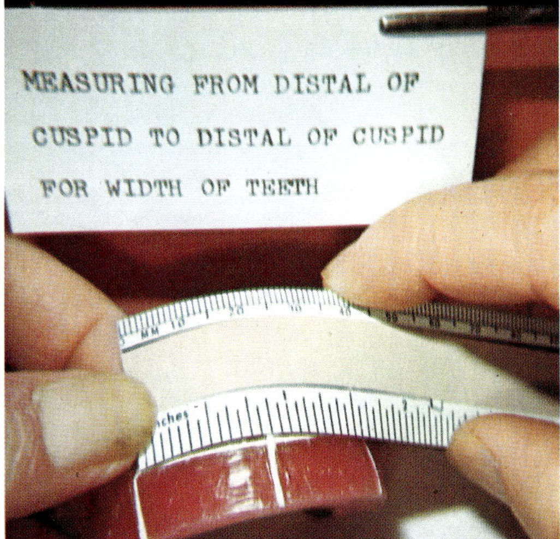

Fig. 11-6

11. Selecting and Setting the Anterior Teeth

There are many methods by which dentists have been selecting and setting anterior teeth. I will illustrate one procedure that should be easy to follow. However, for those who wish to use an alternate approach, I refer them to Chapter 11 in *An Atlas of Complete Denture Prosthesis.*

1. The previously corrected contoured and length-established maxillary wax bite block is reinserted in the mouth (Fig. 11-1).
2. The patient is asked to smile, and the height of the lip line is observed (Fig. 11-2). With the straight edge of a ruler, mark this "smile line" parallel to the incisal aspect of the bite block (Fig. 11-3).
3. Using the ruler, mark the distal of the cuspid areas on the bite block by placing the ruler in line with the lacrimal duct and the ala of the nose on both sides of the face (Fig. 11-4).
4. Mark the medial line (Fig. 11-5).
5. With a ruler measure the distance in millimeters from the distal aspect of the cuspid line on one side to the distal aspect of the cuspid line on the opposite side (Fig. 11-6). This measurement determines the width of the six maxillary anterior teeth.

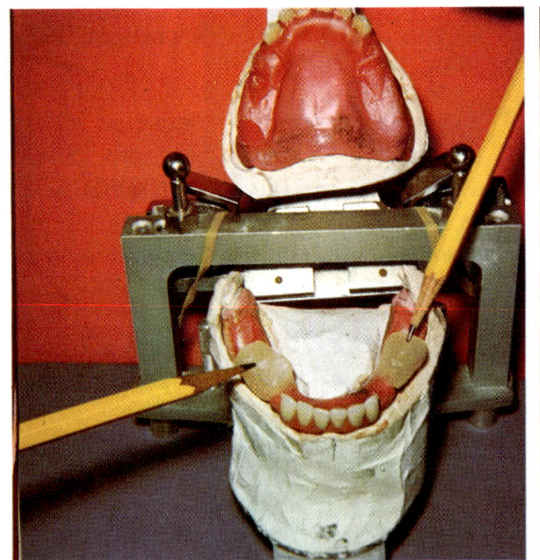

Fig. 12-1

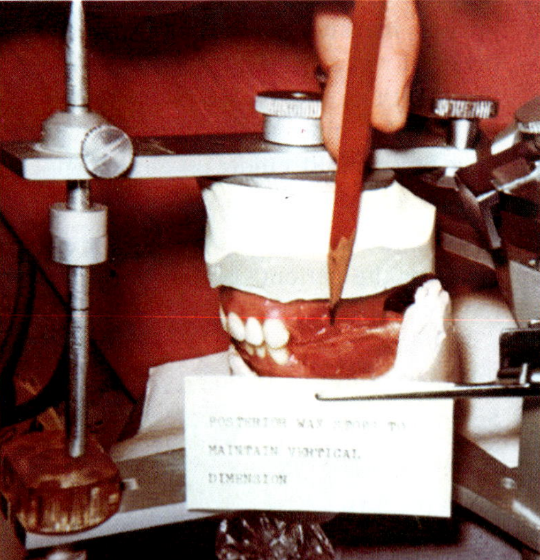

Fig. 12-2

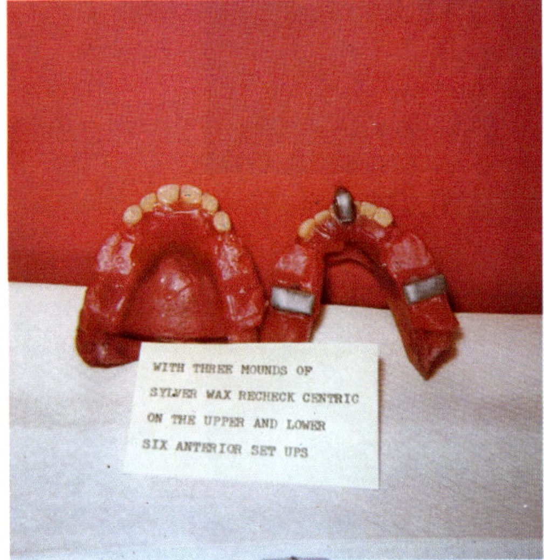

Fig. 12-3

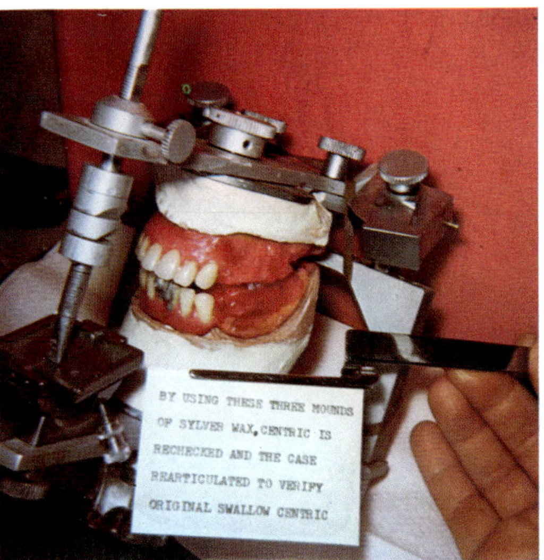

Fig. 12-4

12. Checking Anterior Try-ins for Esthetics and Phonetics

It is best not to finish setting up the posterior teeth at this juncture. I have found that it is easier should corrections have to be made to make sure that the patient and the spouse (whom I insist must be present at the try-in) are completely satisfied with the appearance of the anteriors. Also, if corrections in esthetics are necessary, we avoid resetting the posterior teeth. I also find it easier, without posterior set-ups, to recheck centric occlusion. Therefore, after the six maxillary and six mandibular anterior teeth have been set up, remove the soft wafer swallow-in wax in the molar regions (Fig. 12-1) and substitute hard wax stops (Fig. 12-2) in order to maintain the vertical dimension during the try-in period.

1. With the upper and lower anterior set-ups on the bite blocks we now check for esthetics and phonetics in the mouth.
2. To check for esthetics, insert these bite blocks into the patient's mouth and notice whether the maxillary teeth fall on the inner wet-dry line of the lower lip when the patient pronounces the letter "F."
3. If any deviation is necessary, make corrections.
4. To check phonetics, have the patient count from 60 to 70. When he utters the "S" sound notice whether there is sufficient overjet and that there is no "hissing," that the teeth are not touching, and that they are at least one millimeter apart.
5. Have the patient approve the appearance of the anterior teeth. It is usually essential to have the spouse's approval also.

   If esthetics are satisfactory, it is best at this visit to recheck centric occlusion on these anterior wax try-ins (but first make sure that the musculature is not in spasm).
6. Remove the lower try-in from the mouth and place upon it 3 mounds of laminated wafer wax.*
7. After slightly heating these 3 mounds of wax with an alcohol torch, replace the lower try-in in the mouth, and while gently positioning with the thumb of the right hand—the jaw to the rear-most position—ask him to gradually close until you see that there is slight contact between the 3 mounds of wax.
8. Upon contact, ask him to bring his lips together over the bite blocks. At that moment release your thumb from his chin and ask him to swallow. Have him hold that position and swallow 2 or 3 times every 20 seconds.
9. Thoroughly chill the try-ins with ice water before removing from the mouth.
10. Knock off the original lower cast from the articulator and rearticulate the new swallowed-in try-ins (Fig. 12-4).

*Laminated Wafers, Sylver-Wax. Jac Son Co.

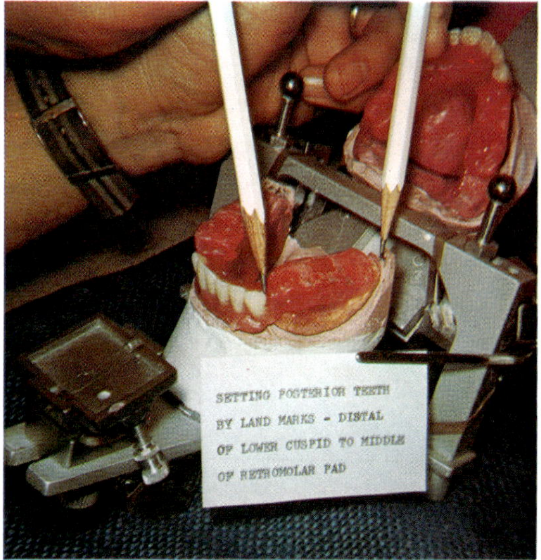

Fig. 13-1

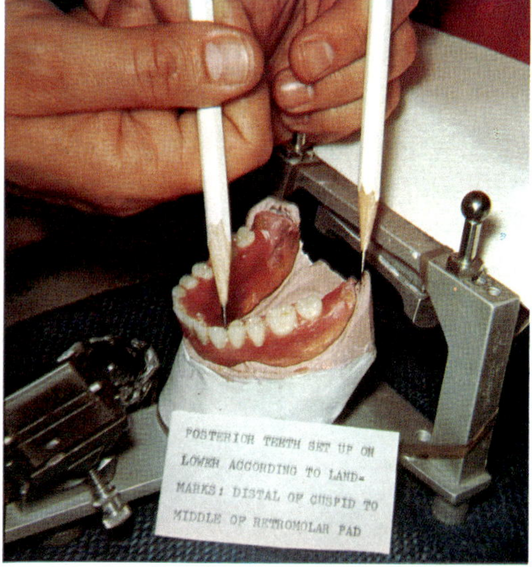

Fig. 13-2

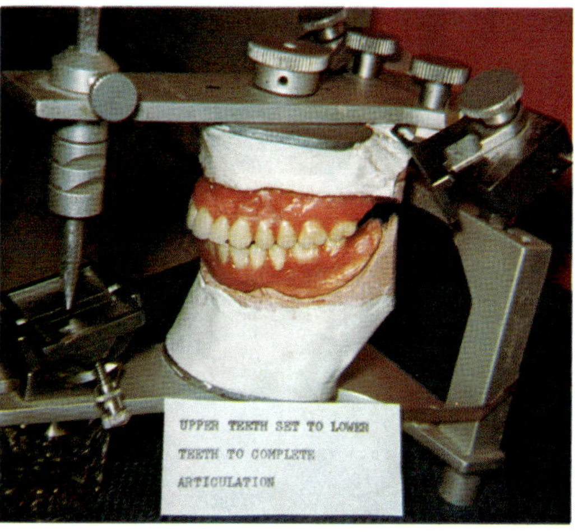

Fig. 13-3

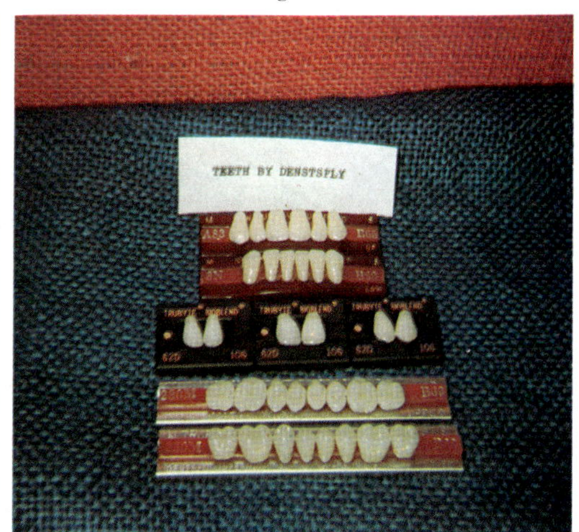

Fig. 13-4

13. Positioning and Setting Posterior Teeth

In a badly mutilated lower jaw, in which most of the landmarks are not present, it is a *must* to make a tongue form in order to set lower posterior teeth in the correct position. (This procedure is described on pages 67 to 70, and pages 86 and 87 in the *Atlas of Complete Denture Prosthesis.*) However, because we are concerned here with the average case, I will describe a simpler method of setting lower posterior teeth by means of landmarks.

1. Mark the middle of the retromolar pad (Fig. 13-1).
2. Set the lower posterior teeth in a virtually straight line, following the

slight curvature upward of the mandible in the molar region from the distal of the cuspid to the middle of the retromolar pad (Fig. 13-2).

3. After completing, by following the landmarks, both sides of the lower posterior set-up, set the upper posterior teeth by articulating them against the lowers (Fig. 13-3).

I use the teeth made by the Dentsply Co.* (Fig. 13-4) almost exclusively because their natural appearance is virtually beyond comparison.

As for their posterior teeth, by using either the Pilkington-Turner or the 33° teeth, I am able to hold the occlusion where I had established it.

*Trubyte Dentsply, Dentsply International.

14. Rechecking Centric Relation and Centric Occlusion on the Completed Wax Set-ups

At this time, after eliminating muscle spasms, recheck by means of wax both centric relation and centric occlusion on the completed set-ups in the mouth. Record the eccentric positions and transfer and incorporate these recordings on the articulator in the following manner:

1. Place 3 mounds of laminated wafer wax on the molar and anterior regions of the mandibular wax try-in denture (Fig. 14-1).
2. Insert the maxillary wax try-in denture in the mouth, first placing petrolatum on the incisal and occlusal surfaces of the teeth.
3. With an alcohol torch, slightly heat the 3 mounds of wax on the mandibular wax try-in denture.
4. Insert that denture in the mouth, and after positioning the jaw, have the patient swallow-in on this wax (Chapter 12, steps 6, 7 and 8).
5. Recheck centric occlusion on the articulator (Fig. 14-2). This recording should match the one done previously.

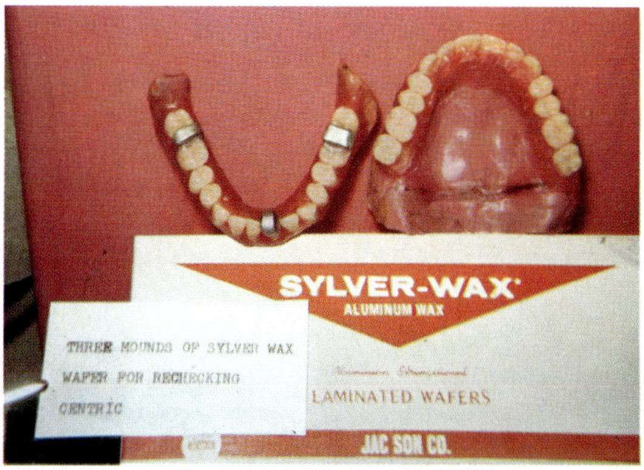

Fig. 14-1

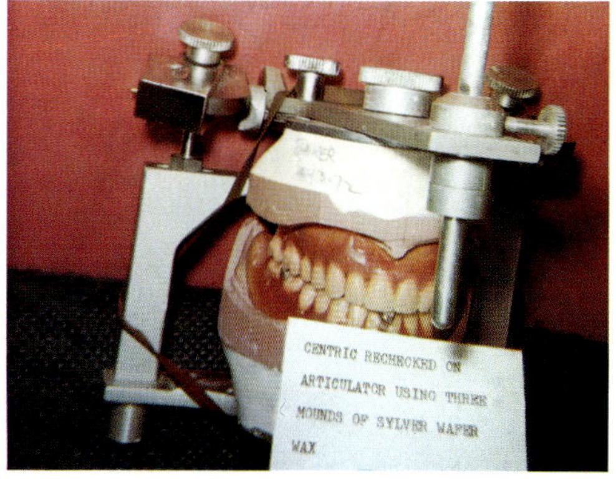

Fig. 14-2

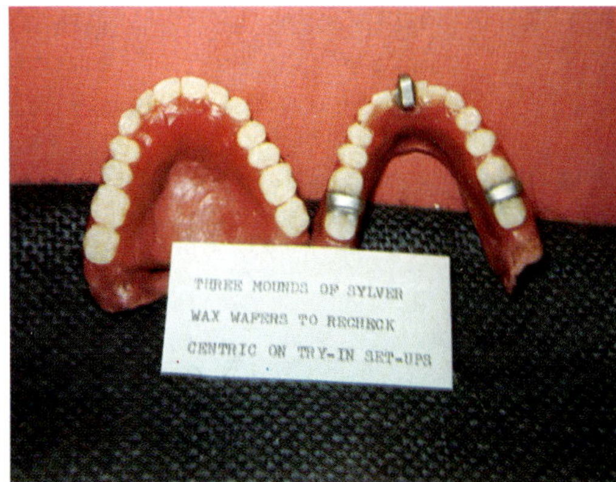

Fig. 15-1

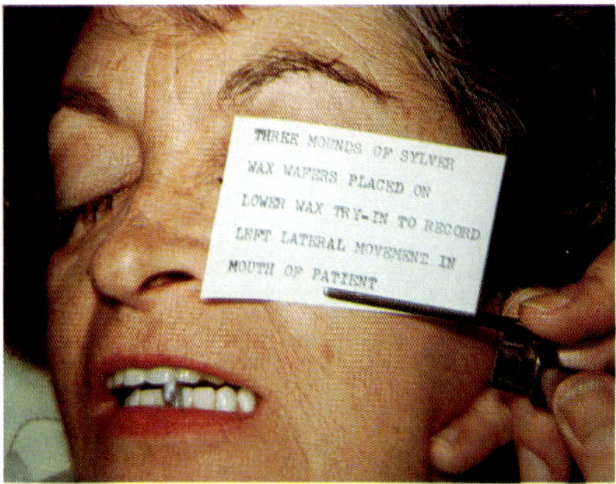

Fig. 15-2

15. Recording the Right and Left Lateral (Bennett Movement) Positions

1. Remove the wax try-in dentures from the articulator.
2. Replace the maxillary try-in denture in the mouth, first placing petrolatum on the teeth.
3. Place 3 mounds of wax on the molar and anterior regions of the mandibular wax try-in denture, as was done for rechecking centric (Fig. 15-1), and heat the 3 mounds slightly with an alcohol torch.
4. Insert the mandibular try-in wax denture in the mouth. After positioning the mandible to the left and while holding that position (Fig. 15-2), ask him to swallow. Thus is the left lateral position recorded.
5. For right lateral position, repeat the same procedure.

16. Setting the Left Lateral Wax Check Bite on the Articulator

1. After removing the left lateral swallowed-in wax try-in denture from the mouth, place it on the articulator.*

   When setting the instrument to the recording, always set the opposite side of the instrument to the side recorded (i.e., if the left lateral check bite position was taken, the right side of the instrument is set).
2. Therefore, since we took the left lateral check bite, ascertain that the ball of the left condyle on the lower part of the instrument is in its socket and that the ball of the right condyle is away from its socket.
3. On the right side, loosen the condyle and Bennett screws.
4. Set the condyle inclination by first

*The Whip-Mix articulator is used throughout this discussion.

tipping the box back and then bringing it down until it contacts the ball on the lower section of the articulator. Tighten the condyle screw while making these adjustments, making certain that the left condyle stays in place and does not move out of position.

5. Take the condylar reading.

6. Adjust the Bennett movement by bringing the lower shift in the box X socket over toward the inside of the articulator first, and then gradually back away toward the outside (or away from the articulator) until the mesial part of the ball is contacted. Lock the screw and record the degree of Bennett movement.

7. For setting the Bennett movement and condylar inclination for the right wax check bite, repeat this procedure on the opposite side of the articulator and record condylar inclination and Bennett movement. (When using the Whip-Mix instrument, protrusive check bites are not necessary.)

For those who do not wish to be so exact, to take lateral wax check bites, I suggest that after centric wax recheck has been taken, set the condylar inclinations at 30° and the Bennetts at 20° on the Whip-Mix instrument and balance the set-up to these positions. The tissue treatment that will be used later on in the procedure will correct the slight differences in the inclinations.

17. Balancing the Wax Dentures on the Articulator

I do not believe that balance on full dentures is a necessity. Then why use balance? Balance is necessary because some patients will inevitably rock their dentures, causing tissue trauma. Since I cannot foretell which patients will suffer this problem, I build a balanced occlusion in all cases, insuring that there is contact at three points when the teeth are in eccentric occlusion. This is done as follows.

1. Move the articulator to one side and make sure that on the working side of the dentition (Fig. 17-1) there is contact on the cuspid and first or second molar, and that on the balancing side there is contact on the first molars.

2. For balancing the opposite side of the detition, repeat step 1, making sure that there is two-point contact on the working side and one-point contact on the balancing side.

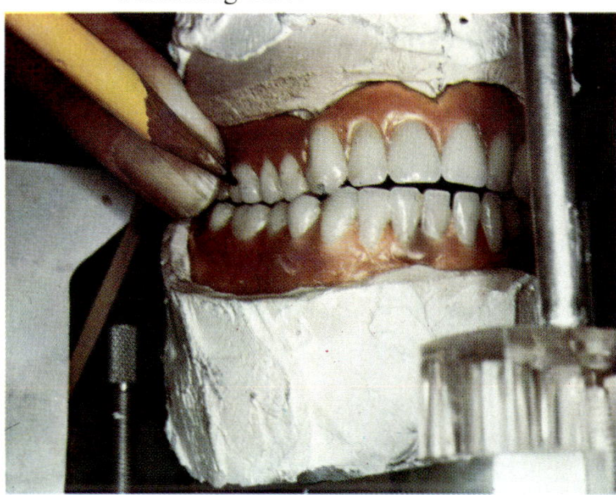

Fig. 17-1

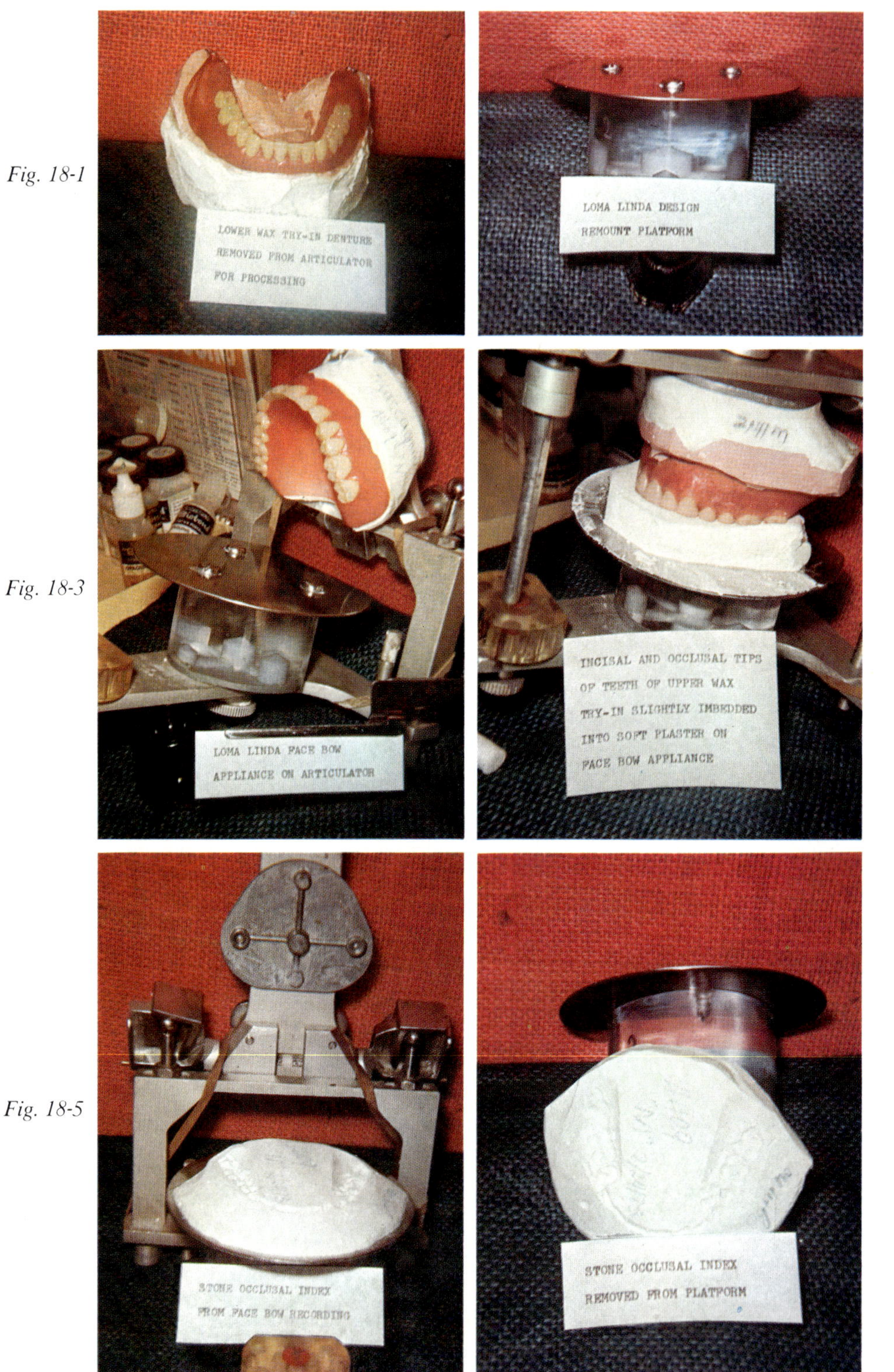

Fig. 18-1

Fig. 18-2

Fig. 18-3

Fig. 18-4

Fig. 18-5

Fig. 18-6

18. Making a Record of the Face Bow Transfer

First, wax down the upper and lower wax try-in dentures to their respective casts on the articulator. Then:

1. Remove the lower try-in denture model and ring, intact from the articulator (Fig. 18-1).
2. A much simpler procedure for making a face bow transfer is now available by using an appliance (Fig. 18-2) developed by Dr. John O. Neufeld at Loma Linda University School of Dentistry. Whip-Mix Corp. also has a somewhat similar appliance. This appliance screws on the bottom part of the articulator (Fig. 18-3) instead of the ring. After mixing and placing fast-set stone on its platform, the upper part of the articulator holding the try-in wax denture is lowered and the teeth indented 1.0 to 1.5 mm. (Fig. 18-4).
3. When the stone index has set, open the articulator. Remove the appliance and stone index intact (Fig. 18-5).
4. Separate the stone index disc from the appliance (Fig. 18-6), mark it with the patient's name and set aside for future use.

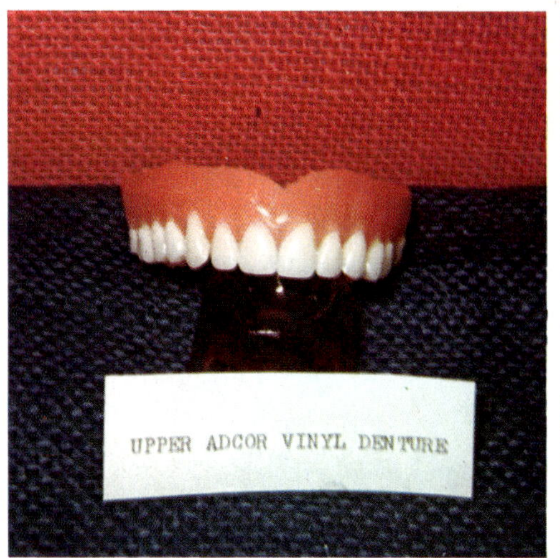

Fig. 19-1

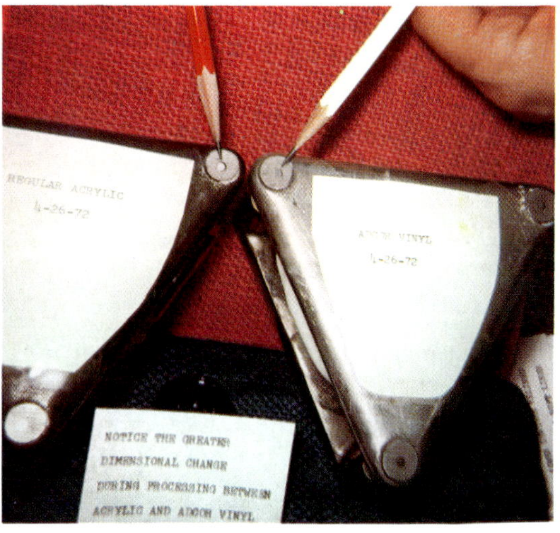

Fig. 19-2

19. Removal of Dentures From the Articulator and Their Dispatch to the Laboratory

Most prosthodontists agree that it is better to process one case at a time. In this manner it is possible to minimize the effect of any changes that take place in the occlusion and elsewhere during processing. Furthermore, it is possible to correct the occlusion by taking a new centric registration in the mouth using the finished maxillary processed denture and the unfinished lower wax try-in denture. If any occlusal adjustments are necessary, they can be made on the articulator before processing the mandibular denture.

1. Therefore, rewax the upper case for processing and remove both cases from the articulator.
2. Send only the upper try-in denture to the laboratory with instructions that it be processed and returned with an upper plaster remount model.

Although there are many acrylics and a few vinyls on the market that offer relatively good strength and quality, I prefer to use Adcor* liquid and powder (Fig. 19-1) because there is practically no odor or water absorption and far less dimensional change during processing (Fig. 19-2), with more tensile strength. This material also has better translucency and more consistent fiber placement, affording better esthetics.

*Adcor, Hard Denture Vinyl. Jac Son Co.

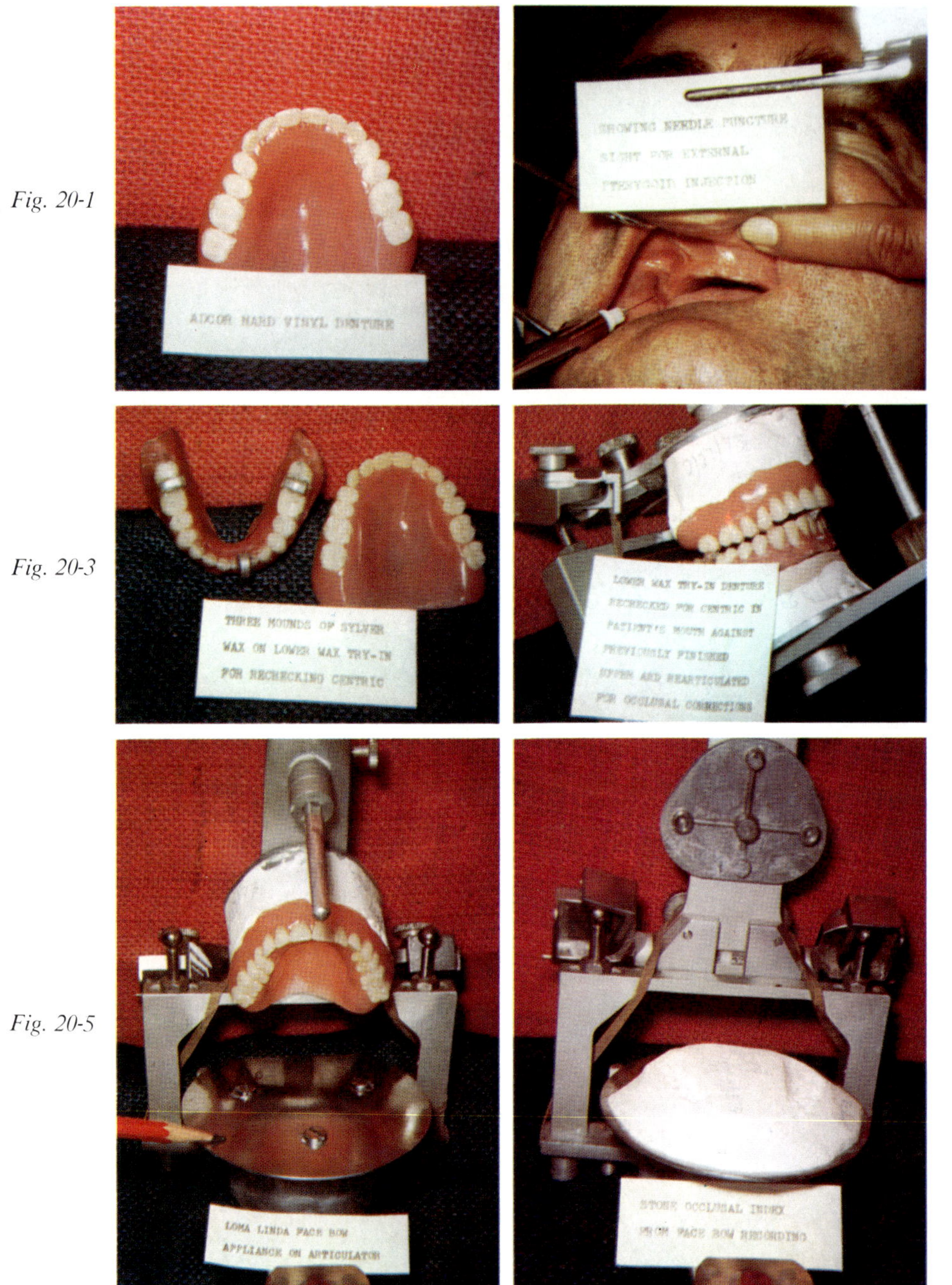

Fig. 20-1

Fig. 20-2

Fig. 20-3

Fig. 20-4

Fig. 20-5

Fig. 20-6

20. Return From the Laboratory of Finished Dentures With the Remount Model

UPPER DENTURES

1. Carefully examine the upper vinyl denture (Fig. 20-1) with the remount model for areas that are rough or sharp.
2. Check muscle spasm and inject spasm areas if necessary (Fig. 20-2).
3. After placing petrolatum over the incisal and the occlusal surfaces of the maxillary teeth, insert the upper finished denture into the mouth.
4. Place 3 mounds of laminated wafer wax stops on the molar and anterior regions (Fig. 20-3) of the lower wax try-in denture.
5. After heating these 3 mounds of wax slightly with an alcohol torch, insert the try-in denture and ask the patient to swallow in as was done in the past.
6. Remove the swallowed-in dentures (Fig. 20-4) from the mouth and articulate. Using the previous face bow appliance record (Fig. 20-5), separate the upper denture from the lower and place the former together with the remount model (Fig. 20-6) into the face

FINISHED DENTURE ON
OCCLUSAL INDEX AND
ARTICULATED

Fig. 20-7

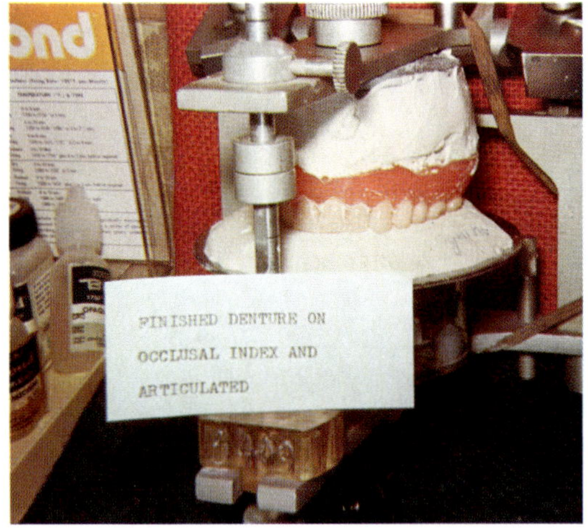

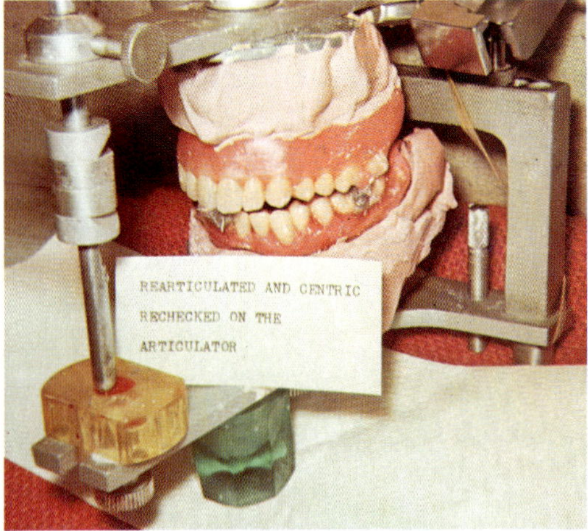

Fig. 20-8

FINISHED DENTURES WITH
REMOUNT MODELS

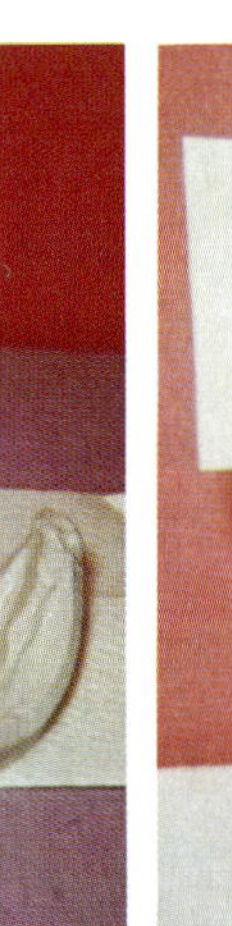

Fig. 20-9

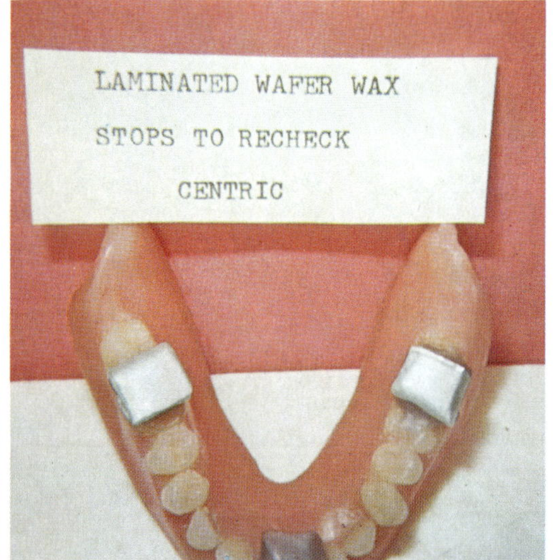

Fig. 20-10

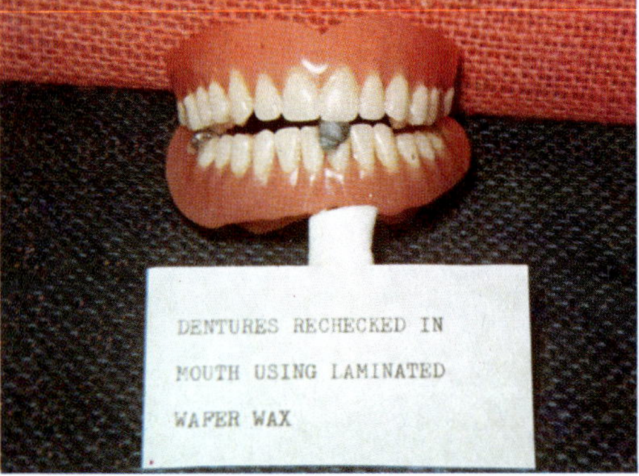

Fig. 20-11

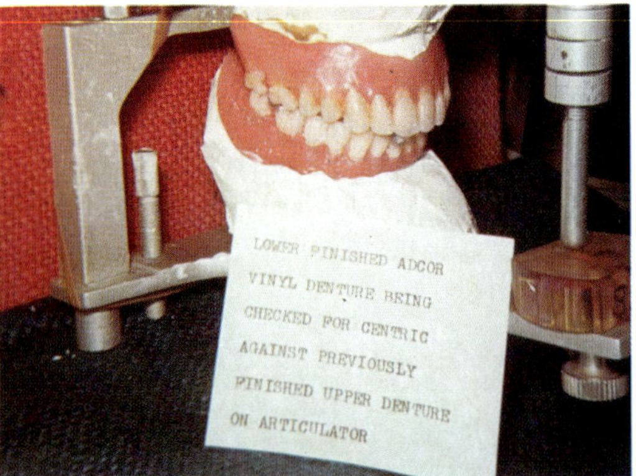

Fig. 20-12

bow record. Attach quick fast-setting plaster to the upper part of the articulator (Fig. 20-7).

7. When the plaster has set, remove the lower face bow recording, and after rechecking centric in the mouth, place a new ring on the lower part of the articulator. Place the lower wax try-in in place on the upper and finish the articulation (Fig. 20-8).
8. Rebalance the occlusion.
9. Rewax the lower try-in denture, remove it from articulator and send it to laboratory (Chapter 19, Step 2).

LOWER DENTURES

1. Carefully examine the completed lower vinyl denture and the upper denture with the remount model on the articulator (Fig. 20-9) for any rough or sharp areas after the latter is returned by the laboratory.
2. Check for muscle spasms and inject if necessary.
3. Remove the upper denture from the articulator, its having previously been oriented to the face bow recording. Place petrolatum on the incisal and occlusal surfaces of the maxillary teeth and insert the upper denture in the patient's mouth.
4. Place 3 mounds of laminated wafer wax on the lower finished vinyl denture (Fig. 20-10).
5. Insert the lower denture in the mouth and ask him to swallow in, as was done previously.
6. Remove the swallowed-in dentures (Fig. 20-11) from the mouth.
7. Transfer these swallowed-in dentures to the articulator. Slide in the lower remount model and finish the articulation (Fig. 20-12) by using fast-setting plaster on the lower part of the articulator ring.

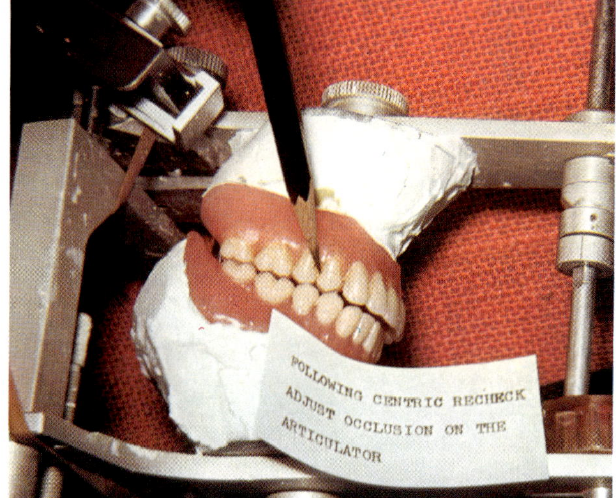

Fig. 21-1

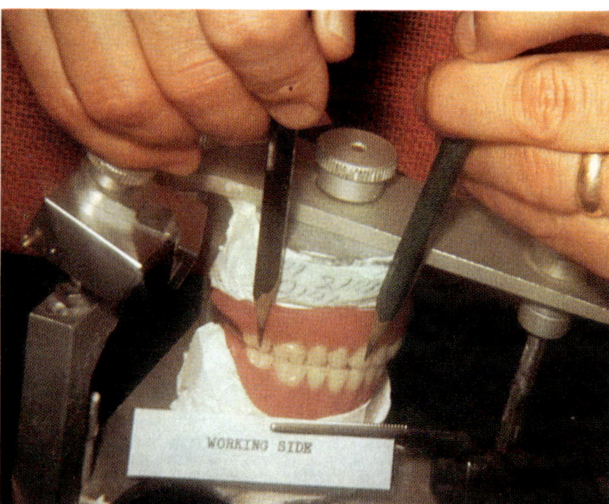

Fig. 21-2

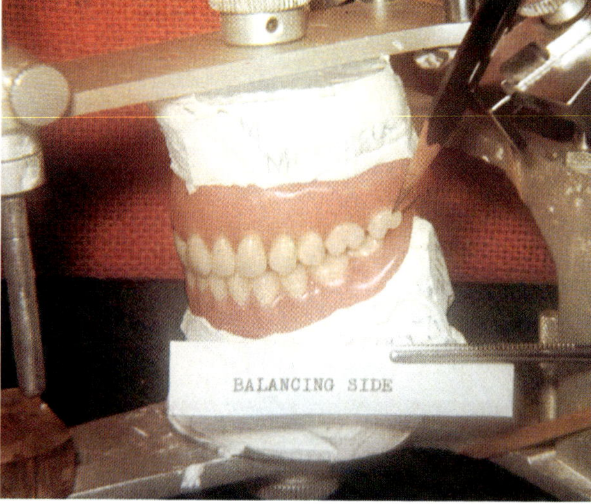

Fig. 21-3

21. Adjusting the Occlusion of the Finished Dentures on the Articulator

After first taking centric check bites in the mouth, balance the dentures by either setting the articulator to the previous lateral recordings, by setting the condylar inclinations at 25 or 30 degrees and Bennett Movements at 20 degrees, or by rechecked with wax in the mouth.

1. Check for prematurities in centric occlusion (Fig. 21-1).

2. Grind away interferences in such a manner that you achieve the same interdigitation of the molars and bicuspids that you had with the adjusted wax try-in dentures.

3. Next, check the right lateral movement. Move the articulator to the right working side in such a way that the right buccal cusp surfaces of the maxillary first or second molar contact the right buccal cusp surfaces of the mandibular first or second molar. Also, the opposing cuspids on the same side should contact (Fig. 21-2).

4. While the instrument is in this position, check the left side (the balancing side) to make sure that the lingual cusps of the maxillary second molar contact the buccal cusps of the mandibular second molar (Fig. 21-3).

   In order to avoid undue trauma to the ridges, since many patients may be doodlers, build in bilateral balance in all dentures.

5. To adjust the other lateral excursion, the articulator is moved to the left. Steps 3 and 4 above are repeated for the two-point contact on the working side and the one-point contact on the balance side.

6. Recheck the case for balances in both centric and eccentric positions.

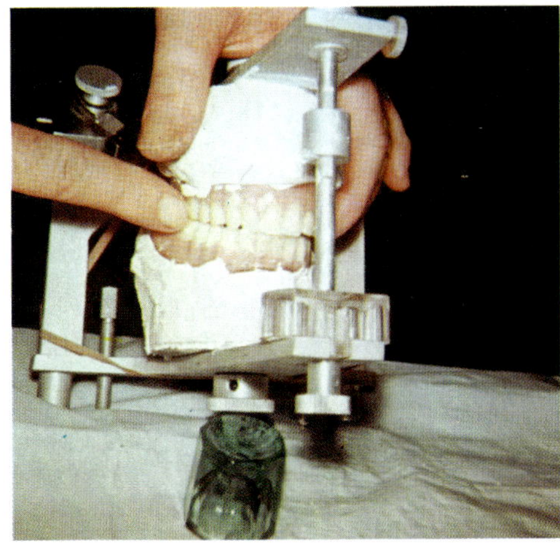

Fig. 22-1

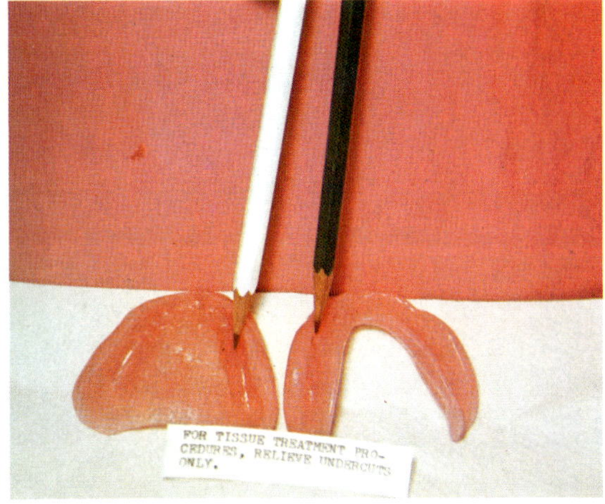

Fig. 22-2

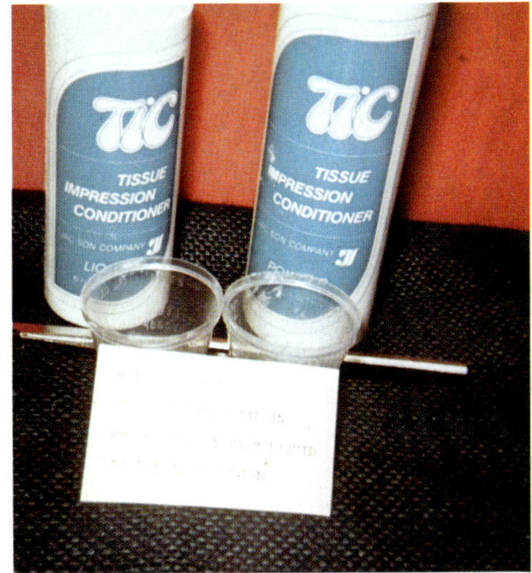

Fig. 22-3

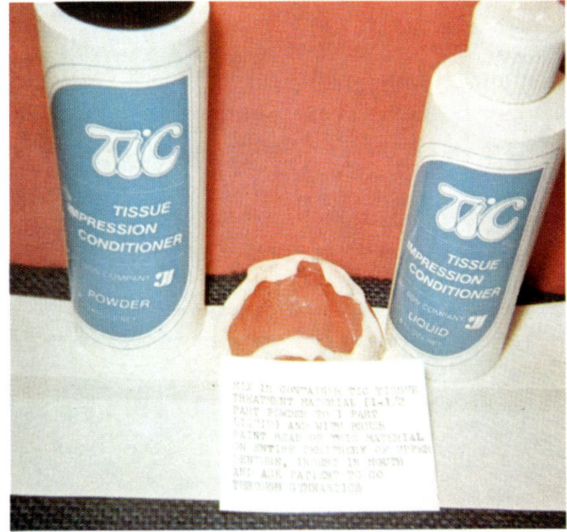

Fig. 22-4

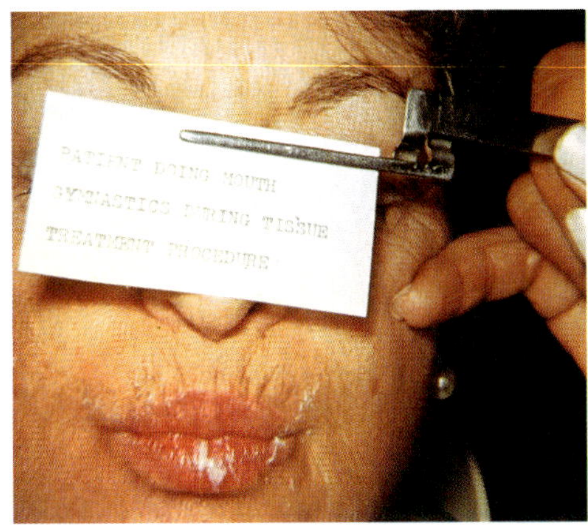

Fig. 22-5

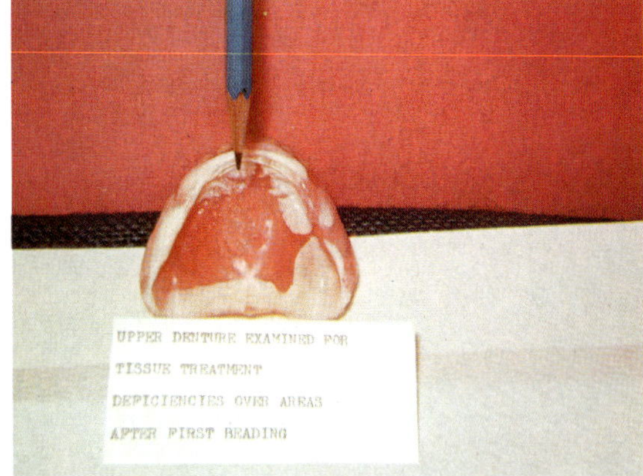

Fig. 22-6

22. Tissue Treatment

All full upper and lower dentures should be fitted with due consideration of the dynamic movements that occur when the wearer actually uses the dentures during talking, chewing and deglutition. Because the original impressions were taken under more or less static conditions (with the least amount of compression), in order to allow for dynamic conditions it is necessary to place tissue treatment under the finished dentures and, following the completion of the treatment process, make these modified dentures permanent for 4 or 5 years by using either a hard vinyl rebase material or a soft cushion material called Adcor Soft Liner.*

When the patient has firm, well-defined, non-resilient and non-pathologic tissue, dentures can be constructed without tissue treatment. However, where tissues have suffered abuse from previous dentures that were ill-fitting, or because of a closed or open vertical, tissue treatment is imperative. Although it is often said that "tissue contained in the denture cannot go anywhere," the displaced and misshaped tissue, when covered by a denture and subjected to the dynamic stress of use, reacts like a sausage-shaped balloon—when pressed at one point it changes shape. Furthermore, upon treating such tissue and comparing the progress models of the jaws from treatment stage to treatment stage, we see that it is not only feasible but essential to return these mouths to normal. If this is not done the patient may never be comfortable. When we observe change in the ridges in many of these cases through the use of comparison photographs of the final treated case and the original, we see tissue that appears not to have come from the same mouth. Let me stress, however, that if sound principles were not applied during construction of the dentures, tissue treatment can do more harm than good.

The patient under treatment should be seen for a change of treatment every 3 days. The length of tissue treatment depends on the condition of the tissue and its severity. The longer the patient has had ill-fitting dentures that have caused considerable displacement and tissue hypertrophy, the longer tissue treatment will take. Cases that are not too severe can be finished (tissue treated) within 1 to 3 visits. Treatment may be required for up to 6 months.

TECHNIC OF TISSUE TREATMENT

I have found in my experience that the newer tissue treatment products work better than others used in the past. TIC† is an example of this because of its smooth texture and longer flow period with greater flexibility. It is now possible to condition a mouth in a fraction of the time it used to take. In some instances with full upper and lower cases, if the tissue on the upper jaw is in good condition, it may be necessary to treat only the lower jaw. However, if both jaws have previously been badly abused, it is necessary to treat both cases simultaneously.

After the laboratory returns the finished cases, and after you have taken new centric records and balanced the cases on an instrument (Fig. 22-1), proceed in the following manner to prepare the dentures to receive the tissue treatment.

1. On the upper and lower, relieve on the inside of the dentures only the vinyl undercuts (Fig. 22-2), nothing else.
2. Using Tic Tissue Treatment† (Fig. 22-3), mix the material—1 part liquid to 1½ parts powder—by spatulating in the container for 20 seconds, to a smooth consistency. Always pour liquid

*Adcor Soft Liner. Jac Son Co.
†Tic Tissue Treatment. Jac Son Co.

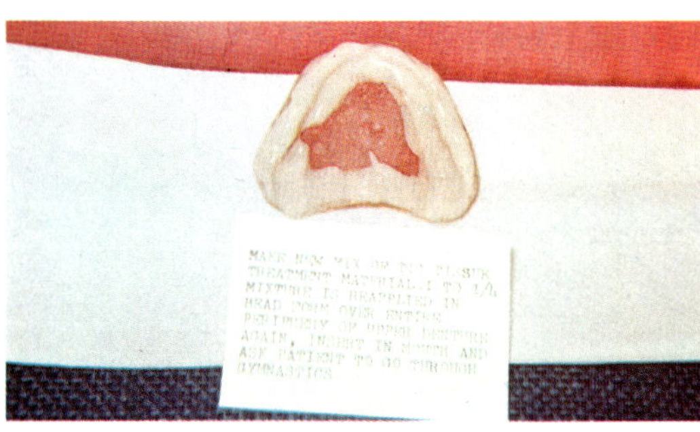

Fig. 22-7

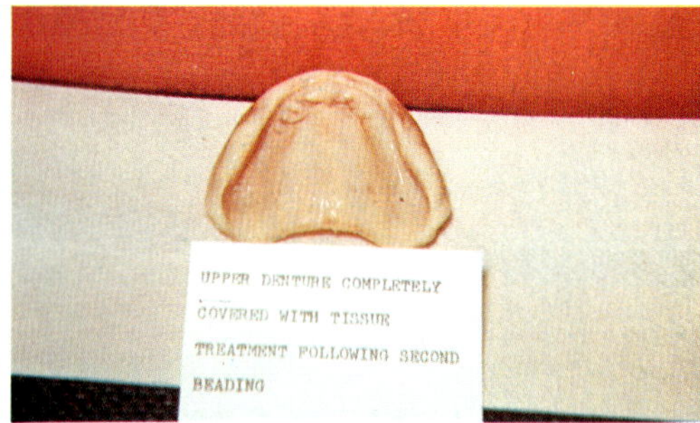

Fig. 22-8

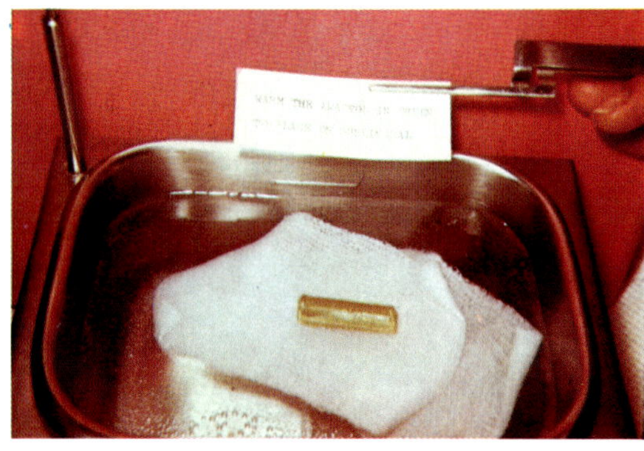

Fig. 22-9

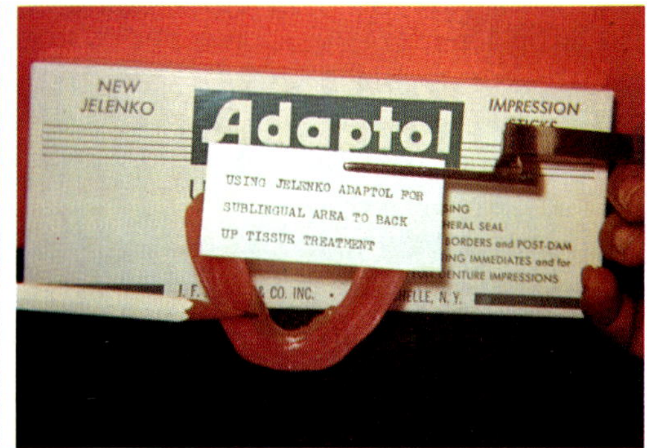

Fig. 22-10

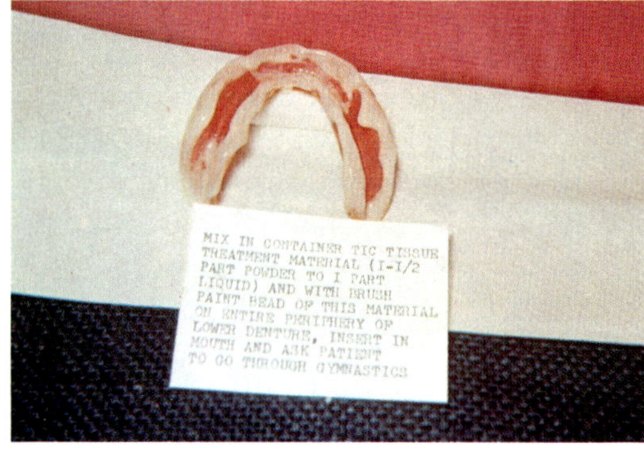

Fig. 22-11

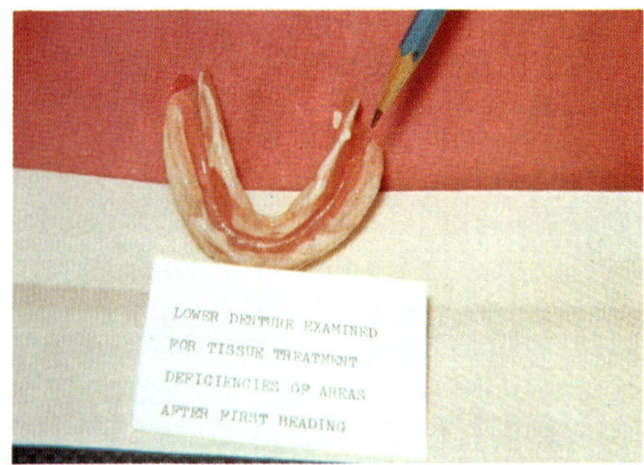

Fig. 22-12

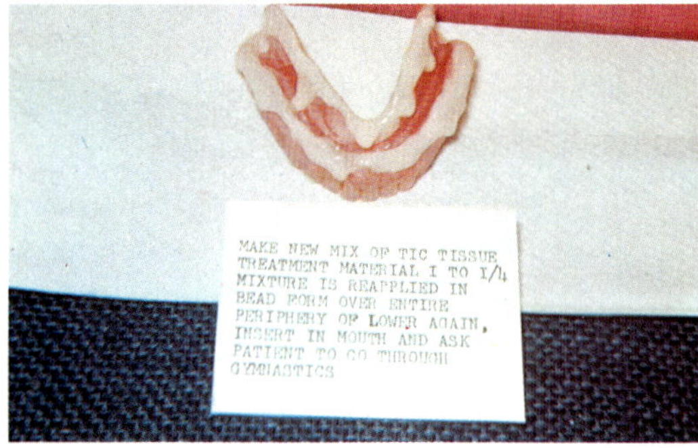

Fig. 22-13

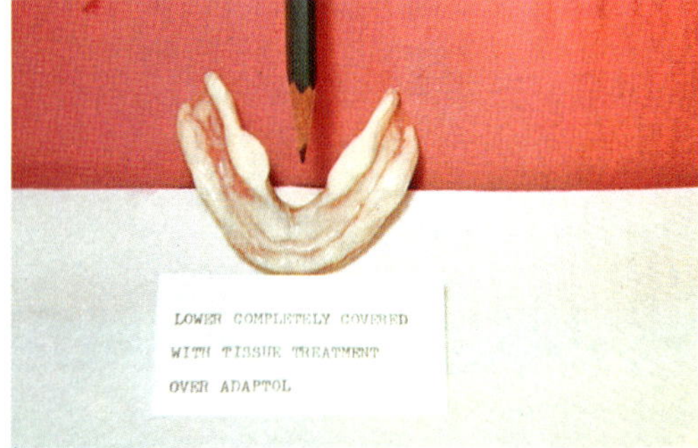

Fig. 22-14

into the container first and then add the powder while constantly spatulating the mixture.

3. Following 20 seconds of spatulation, and with the lower denture in the mouth, immediately begin to paint this tissue treatment material in the form of a bead around the entire periphery of the upper denture (Fig. 22-4) and insert it in the patient's mouth. Ask the patient to bring both dentures together in occlusal contact and begin mouth gymnastics (Fig. 22-5), which consist of puckering, grinning, sucking and swallowing for five minutes.

4. Mouth gymnastics taking place under function cause the tissue treatment material to be sucked into and between the upper denture and underlying tissues without upsetting the occlusion and vertical dimension by more than 0.5 to 0.75 mm.

5. After 5 minutes in the mouth, remove the upper denture and examine for deficiencies in the distribution of tissue treatment material (Fig. 22-6).

6. After drying this partially tissue-treated upper denture with an air syringe, make a new mix of tissue treatment material, this time using 1 part of liquid to 1 ¼ parts powder. Apply this mixture over the entire periphery (Fig. 22-7) and over the previous beaded material.

7. Reinsert the upper denture into the mouth, instructing the patient to assume occlusal contact and go through the mouth gymnastics as was done previously.

8. Following these two paintings with tissue treatment, we usually find that all areas on this upper treated denture are now completely covered (Fig. 22-8). However, if a few spots have been missed in the palatal region, lightly paint over such areas with a fresh one-to-one mixture. Reinsert the denture into the mouth and have the patient hold in occlusal contact for 5 minutes. Gymnastics at this time are not necessary.

9. When the upper denture is satisfactory, remove both dentures from the mouth and trim off any excess tissue treatment material that may have lodged in the occlusal and incisal areas, making sure not to disturb the peripheral roll.

10. Replace the tissue-treated upper denture in the patient's mouth.

11. Place a half stick of Adaptol material* in a water bath (Fig. 22-9), and set at 110°F. to warm the Adaptol for 5 minutes. Place this warmed Adaptol in the sublingual area from the first bicuspid to the first bicuspid of the lower denture (Fig. 22-10). Now slightly heat this area with an alcohol torch. Place the denture in the mouth and ask the patient to close his mouth. After occlusal contact is achieved, instruct him to exert slight pressure with the tongue on the cinguli of the lower lingual surfaces. Remove the lower denture from the mouth and examine the sublingual Adaptol roll. We are now ready to proceed with the tissue treatment of the lower denture.

    After drying the lower denture with an air syringe, mix 1 part of liquid to 1 ½ parts of powder in a container, and paint a bead of the tissue treatment material on the entire periphery of the lower denture, including the area over the Adaptol (Fig. 22-11). Immediately insert in the patient's mouth with the same instructions about occlusal contact. Gymnastics should be performed as was done for the upper denture.

12. After 5 minutes of gymnastics, remove the lower denture from the mouth and examine for tissue treatment deficiencies (Fig. 22-12).

---

*Adaptol Sticks. J. F. Jelenko Co., Inc., New Rochelle, N.Y.

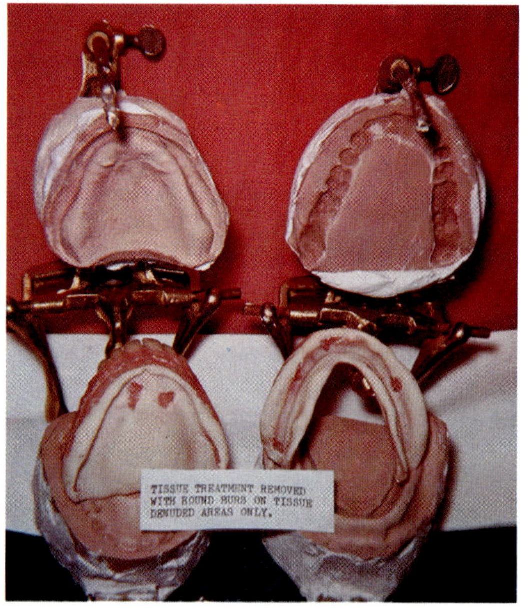

Fig. 22-23

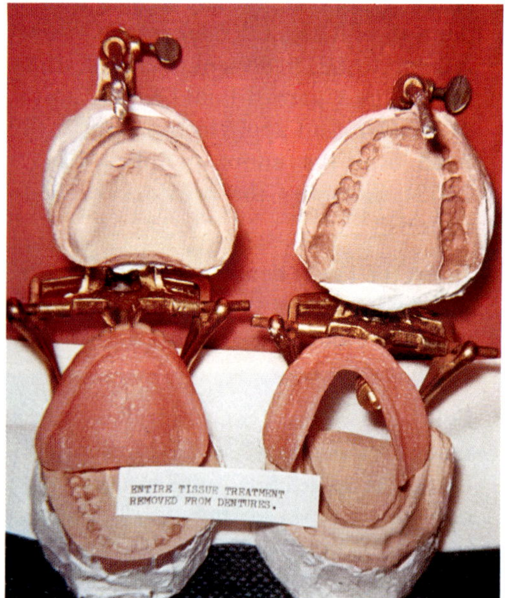

Fig. 22-24

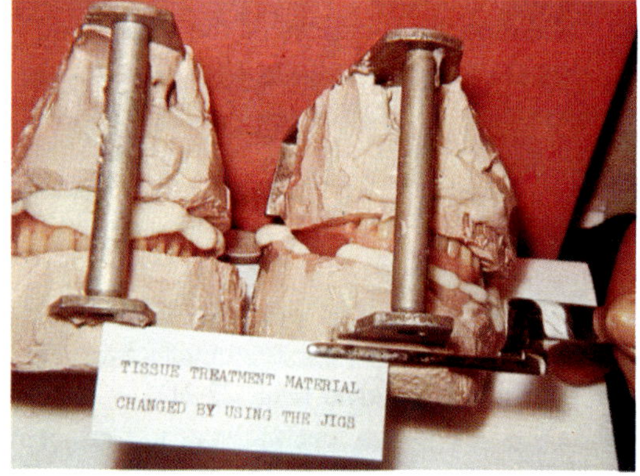

Fig. 22-25

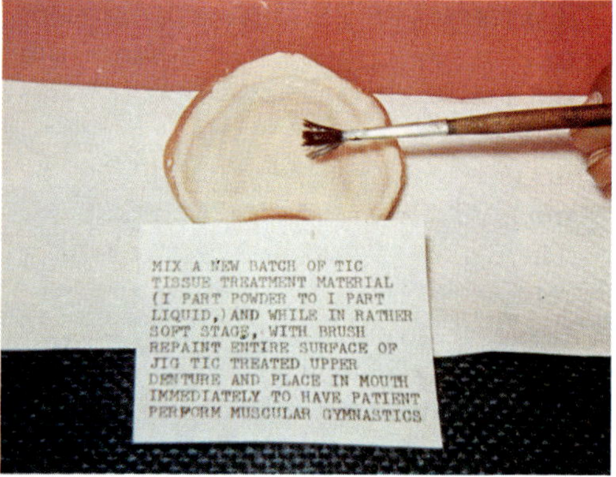

Fig. 22-26

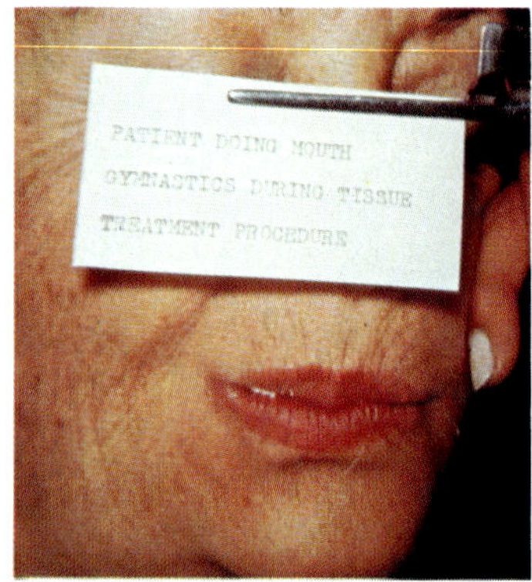

Fig. 22-27

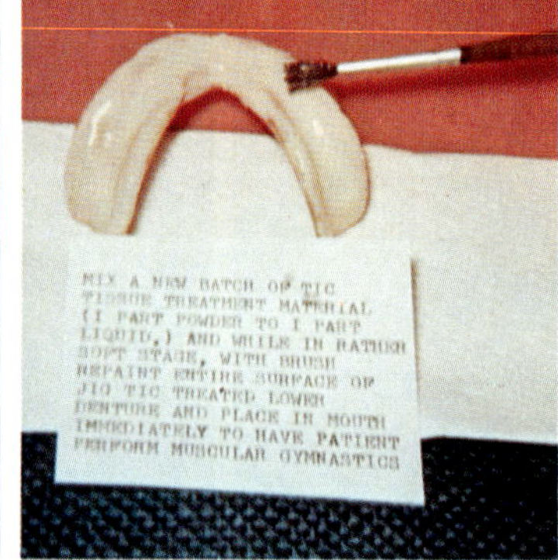

Fig. 22-28

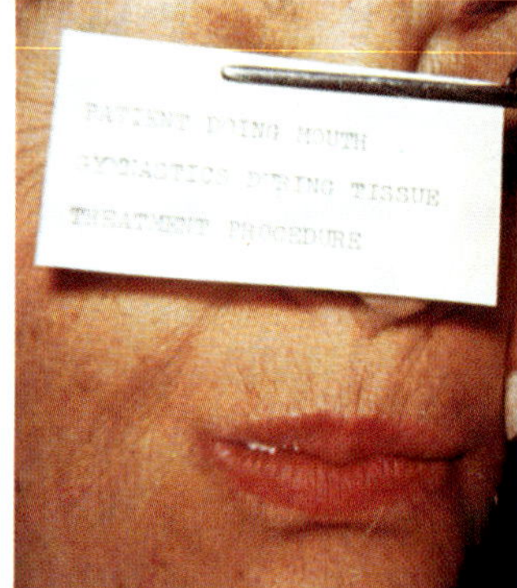

Fig. 22-29

20. With a large round bur, remove the marked denuded areas on the upper and lower dentures (Fig. 22-23).

21. With Kingsley scrapers and a large round bur, remove the remainder of the old tissue treatment material on the upper and lower dentures (Fig. 22-24).

22. Mix the tissue treatment material in the container (1 part liquid to 1½ parts powder). Pour or spread the material into the upper and lower dentures and replace on the jigs (Fig. 22-25). Now place the treated dentures into a container of warm water for 5 minutes to hasten setting.

23. Remove the upper tissue-treated denture from the jig and trim off the excess material.

24. Remove the lower tissue-treated denture from the jig and trim off the excess material

25. Place the lower tissue-treated denture back in the mouth. Mix a new batch of tissue-treatment material (1 part liquid to 1 part powder), and while this is in a soft state, repaint with a brush the entire surface of tissue-treated upper denture (Fig. 22-26). Place this denture in the mouth immediately and ask the patient to come into occlusal contact and then perform muscular gymnastics (Fig. 22-27).

26. After 5 minutes of mouth gymnastics, treat the lower denture in the same manner. While leaving the upper denture in the mouth, remove the lower denture and dry it with the air syringe. Mix a new batch of tissue treatment material (1 part liquid to 1 part powder), and while this is soft repaint the entire surface of tissue-treated lower denture (Fig. 22-28). Place it in the mouth immediately, and after asking the patient to achieve occlusal contact have him perform muscular gymnastics for 5 minutes (Fig. 22-29).

27. After the excess material has been removed, the patient is dismissed and instructed to return 3 days later for a change of tissue treatment.

When the patient returns, if everything is satisfactory, the same jigs are used for changing the tissue treatment. Steps 22 through 26 are repeated. It is necessary for the patient to wear this new change of tissue treatment only over night. When the patient returns the following morning, remove both dentures from the mouth and send them to the laboratory for finalization.

Finalization could involve either a hard rebase material or, better still, one of the recently developed soft reliners.*

*The Adcor Soft Liner. Jac Son Co.

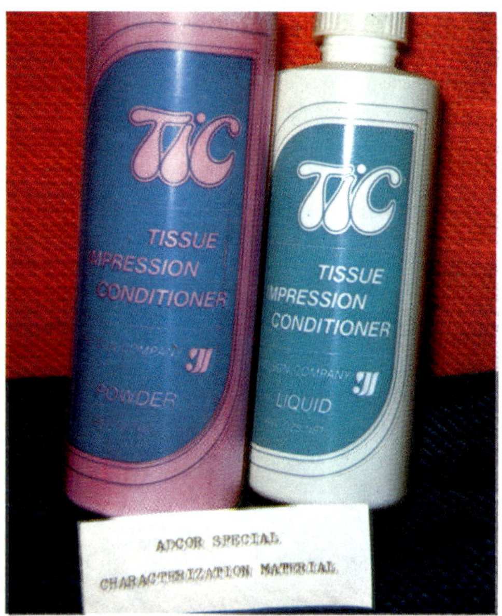

Fig. 23-1

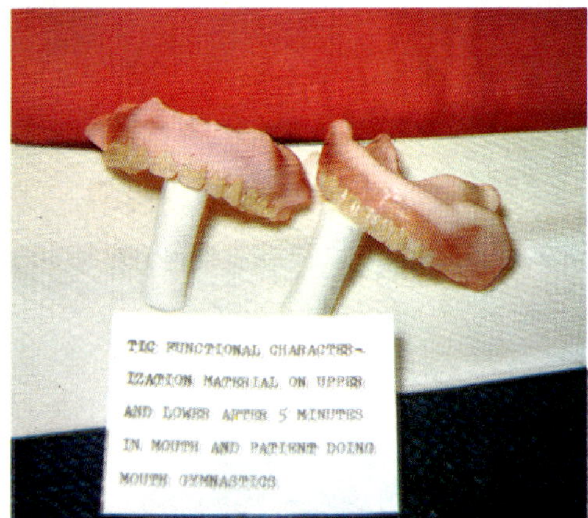

Fig. 23-2

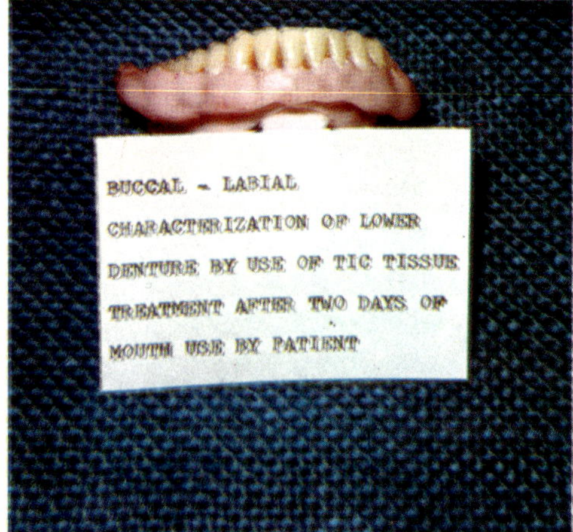

Fig. 23-3

23. Characterization of Dentures

In addition to other benefits, characterization built into dentures can help to improve retention.

For those who wish to achieve complete characterization, I refer them to Chapter 19 in *An Atlas of Complete Denture Prosthesis*. However, for those who wish a shorter method the following efforts will be rewarding:

1. After step 27 in the preceding chapter, and just before the final change of tissue treatment is made on the jigs, thin out the labial and buccal vinyl surfaces of the upper and lower dentures, and instead of replacing with the regular tissue treatment material, place the dentures back on the jig and replace the regular tissue treatment material with tissue characterization material (Fig. 23-1).

2. Follow steps 22 through 27 in Chapter 22.

3. Make a new mix (1½ powder to 1 part liquid) of this tissue characterization material and paint it rather thickly on the thinned down labial and buccal surfaces of both dentures. Replace in the mouth and ask him to go through mouth gymnastics.

4. After 5 minutes of gymnastics, remove the cases from the mouth and examine (Fig. 23-2).

5. Send him home with instructions to return the next morning in order to remove the denture (Fig. 23-3) from the mouth for finalization in either hard material or in a soft liner.

24. Termination of Tissue Treatment

When do you terminate tissue treatment? When the patient is comfortable: when the oral tissues have returned to normal and the patient can use the dentures with maximum comfort and efficiency. The length of time it takes to treat an individual case depends upon the severity of the conditions affecting the oral tissue when the patient first presents for treatment.

In order to achieve the best results you should have the patient return to the office every 3 days in order to change the tissue treatment; after 3 days the tissue treatment material has lost most of its working flow and not only may cause irritation, but, more important, is no longer helping to restore the oral tissues to a normal state. The minimum course of tissue treatment requires 1 to 3 changes of material during treatment. It may also be necessary to check and adjust the occlusion several times. Occlusal discrepancies may occur, especially if there were severe muscular spasms of long duration, causing rotation. Any rotation causes a horizontal rather than an anteroposterior change in occlusion. This can be corrected by use of wax check bites, implementing the Whip-Mix articulator in which a face bow was employed. Another way to correct the occlusion is to use the Baptist Intra-Oral, Extra-Oral apparatus* (fully described on pages 72 and 73 of *An Atlas of Complete Denture Prosthesis*). It should be remembered that the extent of the horizontal mandibular change influences the duration of tissue treatment. However, once all the structures of the stomatognathic system return to normal—especially when the correct vertical and centric relations have been established—the tissue responds faster and the patient is comfortable with the efficient function of his dentures.

*Victor Baptist, 85 Leeuwarden Rd., Darien, Conn. 06820

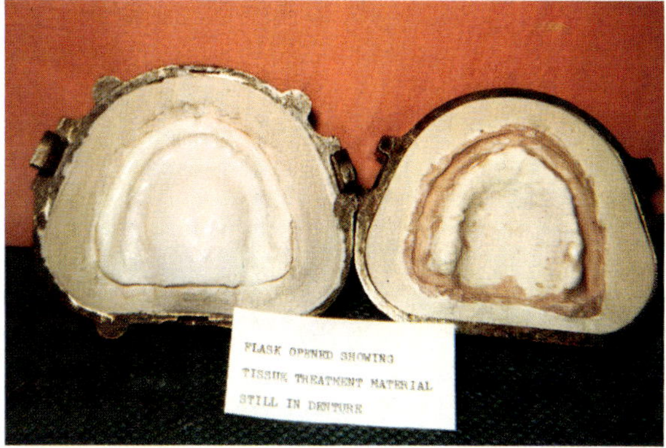

Fig. 25-1

25. Duplicating the Treated Denture Bases After Final Tissue Conditioning

1. The upper tissue-treated vinyl denture (Fig. 25-1) may be rebased by using the regular hard Adcor vinyl material or any good heat cure acrylic in the same manner as is done in an acrylic rebase. However, if the dentist prefers, this upper tissue-treated denture may be rebased with a soft denture liner.*
2. The lower tissue-treated vinyl denture is best treated by using the soft liner.

---

*Adcor Soft Liner. Jac Son Co.

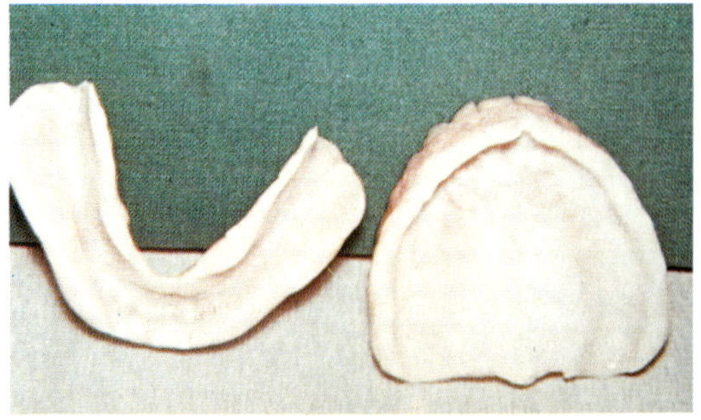

Fig. 26-1

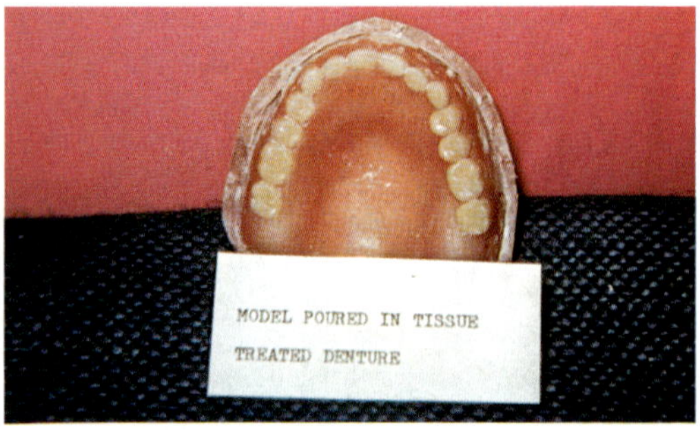

Fig. 26-2

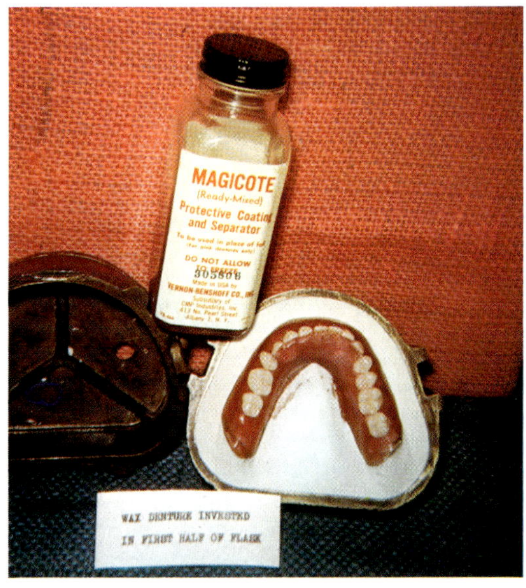

Fig. 26-3

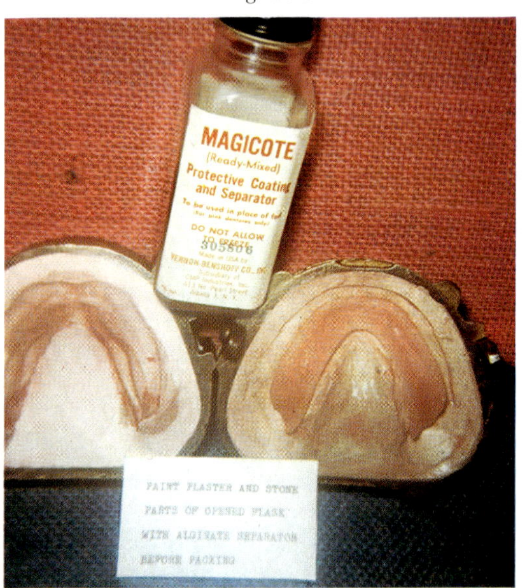

Fig. 26-4

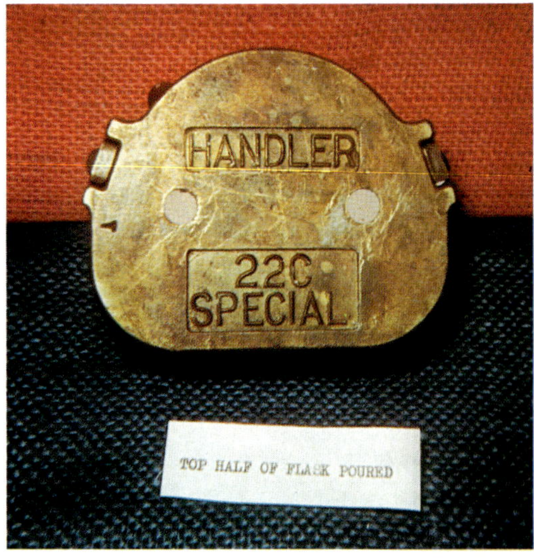

Fig. 26-5

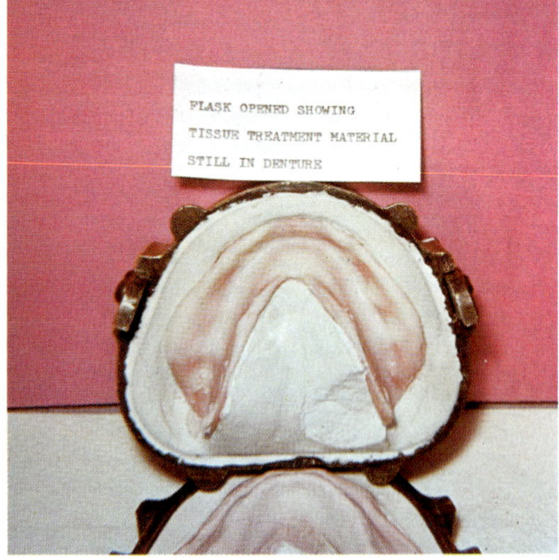

Fig. 26-6

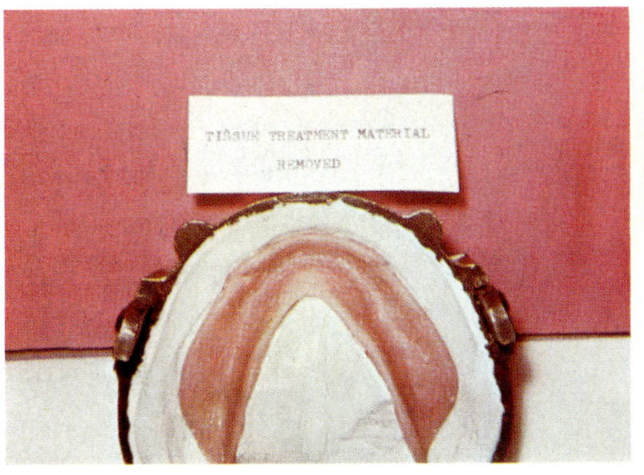

Fig. 26-7

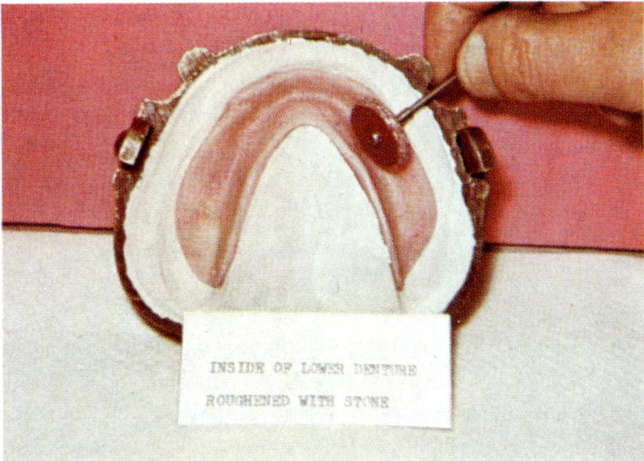

Fig. 26-8

26. Rebasing Tissue-treated Dentures Using Adcor Soft Liner

Whether we use Adcor* soft liner as a cushion rebase on the lower or the upper tissue-treated denture or on both, the procedure is the same.

1. Remove from the mouth the upper and lower tissue-treated dentures (Fig. 26-1) that are to be rebased with soft liner.
2. Pour casts into these tissue-treated dentures (Fig. 26-2) using a good stone composition.
3. Invest in the lower half of the knock-out flask* (Fig. 26-3) using regular plaster.
4. When the plaster has set, paint the plaster area with Adcor Separator* or a good alginate separator (Fig. 26-4).
5. Pour the second half of the flask (Fig. 26-5) using ½ plaster and ½ stone.
6. After the plaster-stone mixture has set, heat the flask in boiling water for 4 to 6 minutes and then slightly tap the flask on the side with a mallet, opening the two halves of the flask and thus exposing the tissue treatment (Fig. 26-6) still in the denture.
7. With Kingsley scrapers and large round burs, remove the tissue-treatment material (Fig. 26-7).
8. Remove with a large round bur and heatless stone about 1.5 mm. of the hard vinyl material from the denture. Grinding the peripheral edge flat at right angles to the buccolabial and the lingual sides of the flange. This allows easy polishing and a smooth invisible line at the seal on either vinyl Adcor* or acrylic denture bases. Finish the now prepared denture by roughening the surface slightly more with a red semi-rough stone (Fig. 26-8), making sure the roughened area includes the entire periphery.

---

*Adcor Soft Liner & Adcor Separator Material. Jac Son Co.

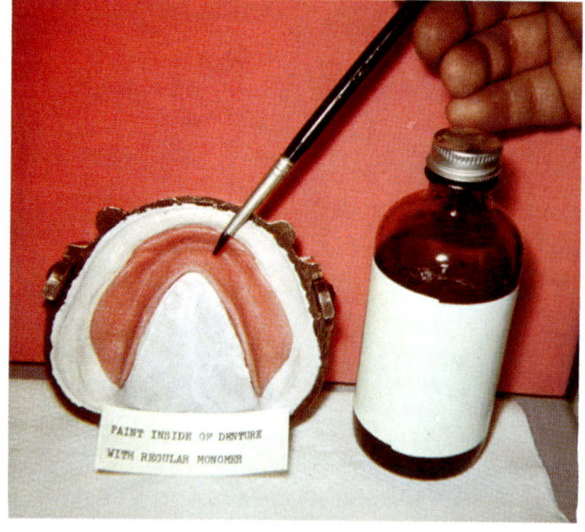

Fig. 26-9

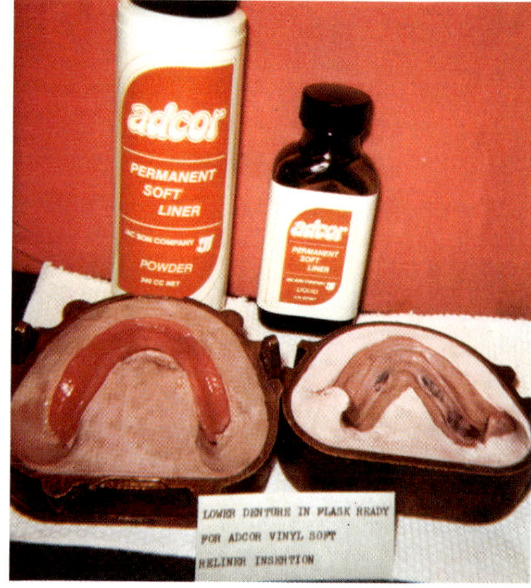

Fig. 26-10

ADCOR SOFT LINER
MIXED IN JAR

Fig. 26-11

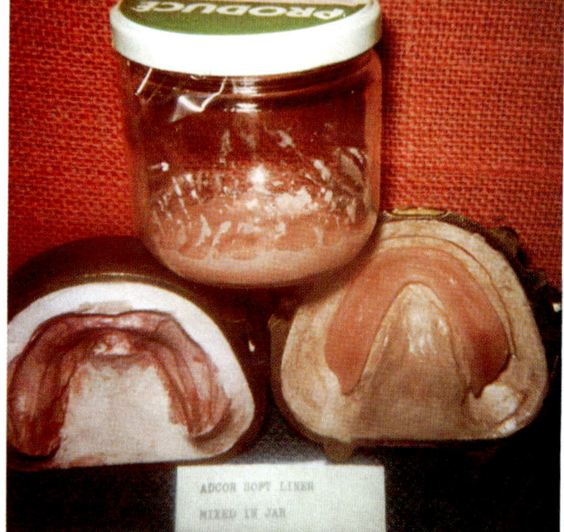

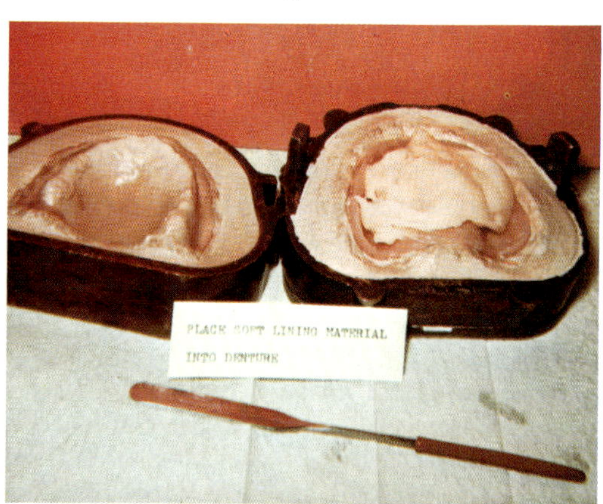

Fig. 26-12

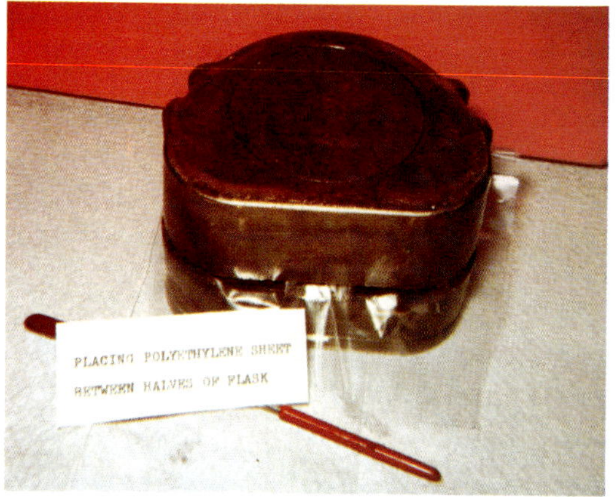

Fig. 26-13

TWO HALVES OF FLASK CLOSED
LIGHTLY WITH POLYETHYLENE
SHEET BETWEEN IN BENCH
PRESS FOR FIVE MINUTES

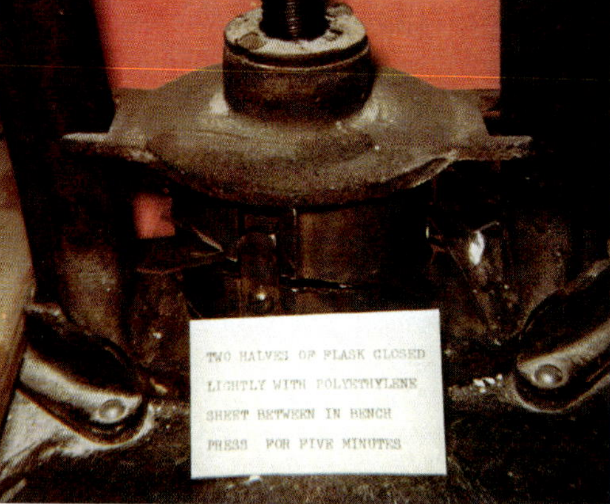

Fig. 26-14

9. Cleanse the denture thoroughly with clean boiling water to eliminate any and all vinyl or acrylic shavings. Apply, according to manufacturer's instructions, a thorough coat of Adcor Separator or a good alginate separator to both stone and plaster areas, allowing separator to dry 5 to 7 minutes until glaze appears, and check for thorough coverage before packing. Paint the inside of the denture with any monomer (Fig. 26-9). The lower denture is now ready for soft liner packing (Fig. 26-10).

10. Mix enough soft liner for the case in a clean glass jar (Fig. 26-11), using exact proportions of 3 parts powder to 1 part liquid (by volume, not weight), tapping powder lightly while measuring, 18 cc. powder to 6 cc. liquid is usually enough for the average case. The setting time before usage of the mixed material should be not less than 20 minutes and should not exceed 30 minutes. Mix should be a little tacky.

11. Pack this soft liner material into the denture (Fig. 26-12), making sure to use cotton pliers to pick up the material. (The moisture of your fingers may contaminate it.)

12. Place a dry polyethylene sheet* (never use wet cellophane or plastic) between the flask (Fig. 26-13), and bring the 2 halves of the flask together.

13. Place the flask in bench press (Fig. 26-14) and close very slowly, keeping under gradual pressure until metal-to-metal contact is achieved. After metal-to-metal contact, hold in press, under pressure, 3 to 5 minutes before opening. This usually takes about 15 minutes.

---

*Polyethylene Sheet (Plastipac). Yates Mfg. Co., 1615 W. 15th St., Chicago, Ill. 60608

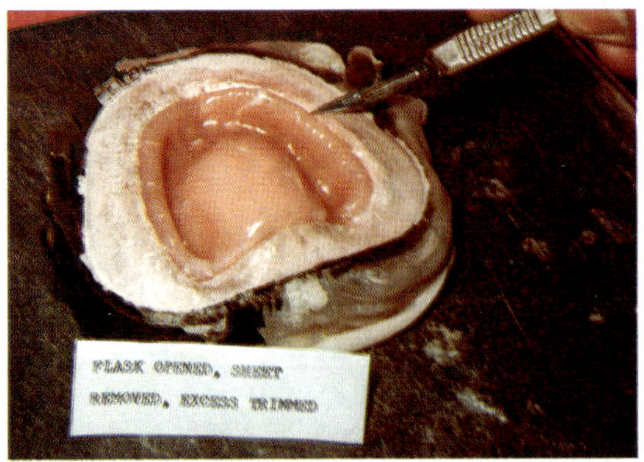

Fig. 26-15

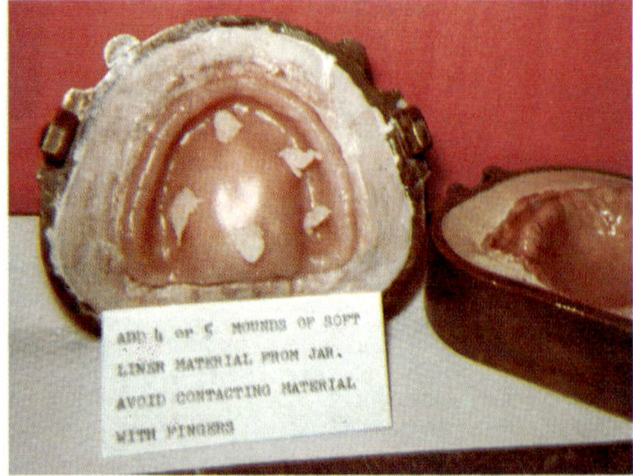

ADD 4 or 5 MOUNDS OF SOFT
LINER MATERIAL FROM JAR.
AVOID CONTACTING MATERIAL
WITH FINGERS

Fig. 26-16

Fig. 26-17

FLASK IS NOW COMPLETELY
CLOSED

Fig. 26-18

PLACE FLASK IN SPRING PRESS
FOR PROCESSING

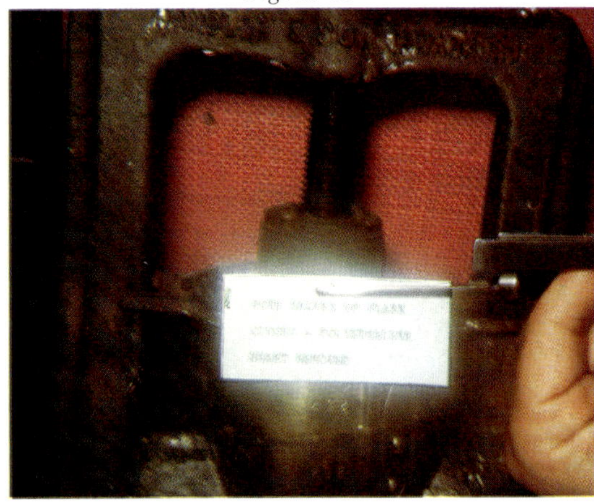

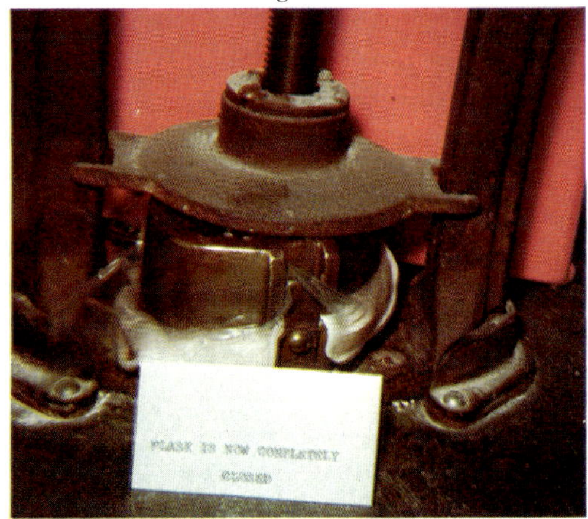

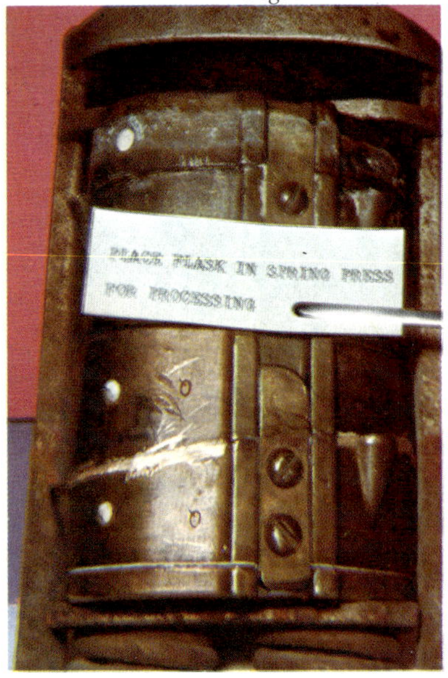

Fig. 26-19

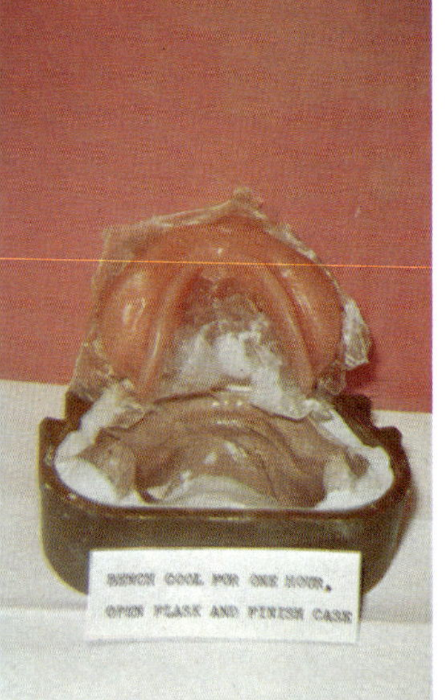

Fig. 26-20

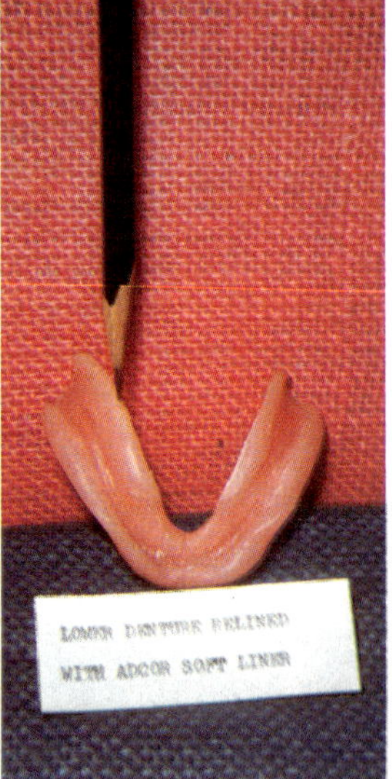

Fig. 26-21

14. Open the flask, remove the polyethylene sheet, and with a Bard-Parker knife trim away the excess (Fig. 26-15).

15. Add 4 or 5 mounds of the soft liner material from the jar (Fig. 26-16), avoiding finger contact.

16. Close both halves of the flask, with no polyethylene sheet between the halves, and place in bench press for final closure (Fig. 26-17). Apply slow and gradual pressure until metal-to-metal contact, leaving in the press under pressure for at least 10 minutes and preferably 20. This usually takes from 20 to 30 minutes.

17. Trim the excess (Fig. 26-18), remove from the bench press, and place in spring press (Fig. 26-19) to be cured in an opened thermostatically controlled water bath.

18. The curing is accomplished by 2 methods.

    FAST CURING: Place case in room temperature water and raise temperature to 165°F (74°C). Leave at 165°F (74°C) for 1½ hours, raise to boil for 1 hour. Allow to bench cool at least 30 minutes and then cool for 20 minutes under tap water.

    OVERNIGHT CURING: Place case in room temperature water, raise temperature to 165°F (74°C) and cure for a minimum of 12 hours. Allow to bench cool at least 30 minutes and then cool for 20 minutes under tap water.

    For added patient comfort if the case is raised to a boil before removing, this will evaporate 2 per cent of the remaining 3 per cent monomer.

19. Open the flask, remove and separate the soft lined case (Fig. 26-20) from the stone casting, and plaster, trim and polish in the normal manner.

20. A finished soft relined denture (Fig. 26-21).

Because new material was introduced in the form of a rebase, to finalize the tissue-treated denture the occlusion must be rechecked under the same conditions as when it was checked originally.

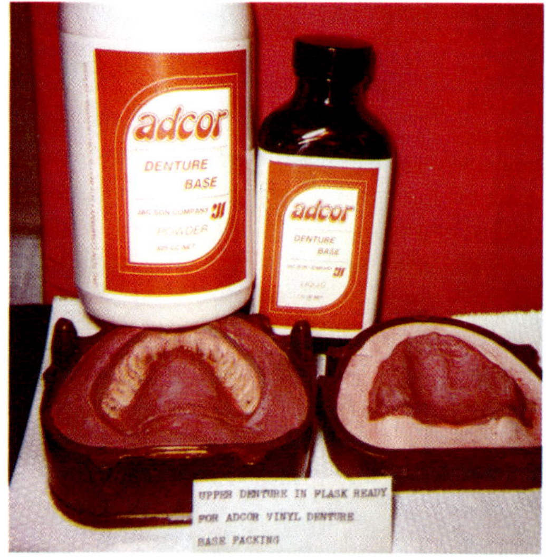

Fig. 27-1

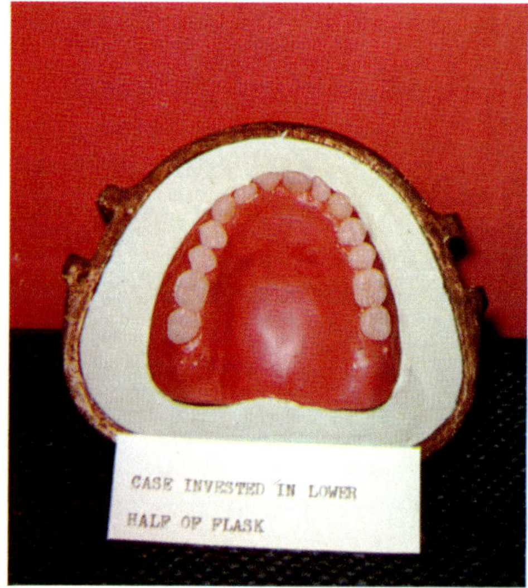

Fig. 27-2

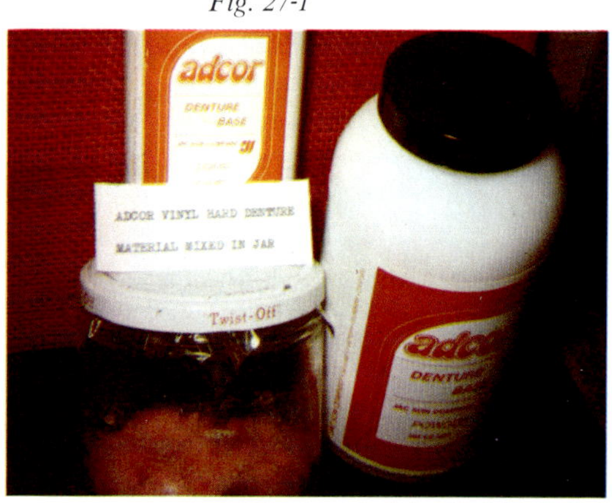

Fig. 27-3

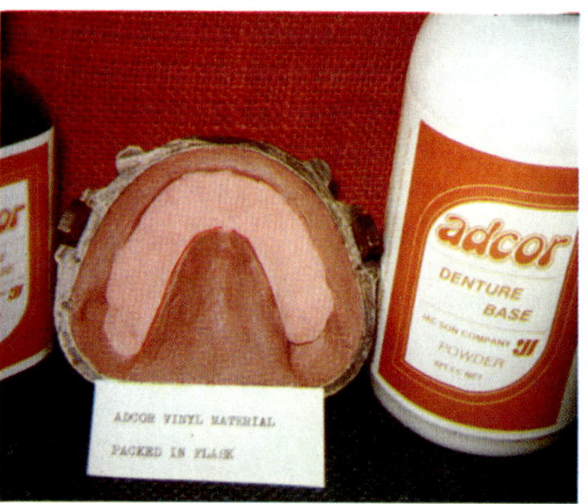

Fig. 27-4

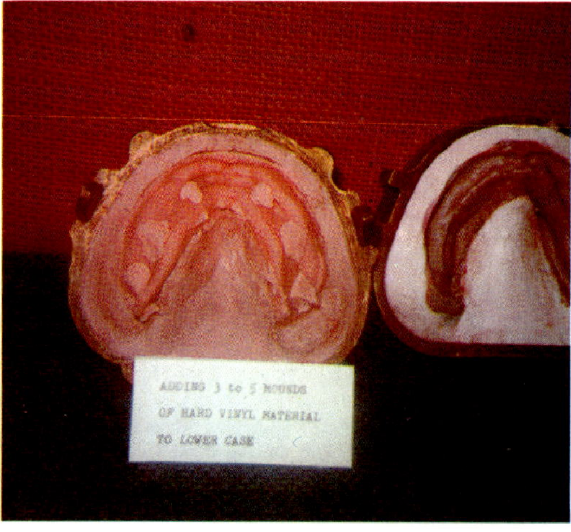

Fig. 27-5

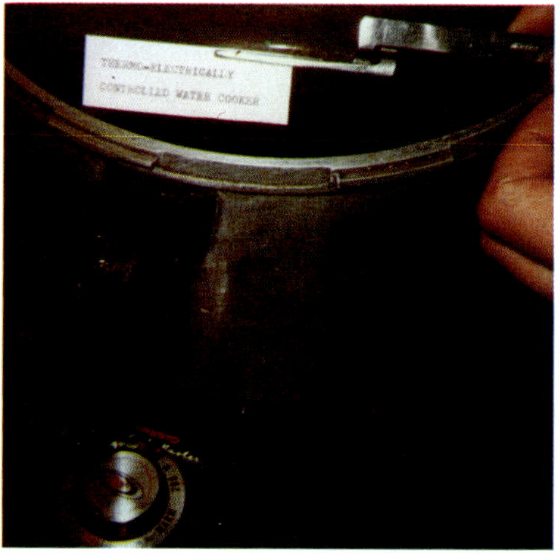

Fig. 27-6

27. The Hard Vinyl Denture Technic Using Adcor Denture Base Material (Fig. 27-1)

1. Invest, by using a good mix of plaster, the upper wax try-in denture in the lower half of the knock-out flask* (Fig. 27-2).

2. After applying Adcor Separator,† a good alginate separator or petrolatum to the plaster investment, pour the upper half of the flask using a mixture of ½ stone and ½ plaster.

3. When the stone and plaster investment has set, place the flask in boiling water for 6 minutes to soften the wax.

4. Remove the flask from the boiling water and, with the slight tap of a mallet, open up the 2 parts of the flask.

5. With a ladle using boiling water, thoroughly flush out the wax after first removing the shellac tray.

6. While the two halves are still warm apply, according to manufacturer's instructions, a thorough coat of Adcor Separator* or a good alginate separator over both halves of the flask and permit to soak for 3 minutes before washing off the excess of material with cold water.

7. Set flasks on their sides to allow excess water and separator material to dry (10 to 15 minutes).

8. The case is now ready to be packed with Adcor Vinyl Material* (Fig. 27-3). The proportions of slightly over 3 parts powder to 1 part liquid (by volume, not weight), tapping powder lightly while measuring, 32 cc. powder to 10 cc. liquid is usually enough for an upper case. This mix should be a bit drier than mixes of acrylic material.

9. Mix the powder and liquid in a glass container and let it sit for 20 minutes. This material or any left-over portion may be stored in a closed jar in the refrigerator for future usage. Many laboratories premix the material and leave in a closed jar in the refrigerator overnight or for future usage.

10. Now pack the vinyl material into the flask (Fig. 27-24). If preferred the material may be worked as dough and shaped like a horseshoe while packing. Place a polyethylene sheet over the material (never use wet cellophane or plastic); bring the other part of the flask over the top, place in a bench press and close slowly, keeping under gradual pressure until metal-to-metal contact is achieved.

11. After the flask is completely closed, remove the flask from the press, open the flask, remove the polyethylene sheet and trim away the excess material.

12. Add 3 or 4 mounds of vinyl material (Fig. 27-5) to the case and close the flask omitting the polyethylene sheet. Place in bench press and apply slow and gradual pressure until metal-to-metal contact. Leave in press, under pressure, 10 minutes before curing.

13. Remove the flask from the press and place in spring press for curing.

14. The curing is accomplished by 2 methods.

    FAST CURING: Place case in room temperature water and raise temperature to 165° F (74° C). Leave at 165° F (74° C) for 1½ hours, raise to boil for 1 hour. Allow to bench cool at least 30 minutes and then cool for 20 minutes under tap water.

    OVERNIGHT CURING: Place case in room temperature water and raise

---

*Controlled water bath unit. Coe Laboratory Co., Chicago, Ill.

†Adcor Denture Base Material & Adcor Separator Material. Jac Son Co.

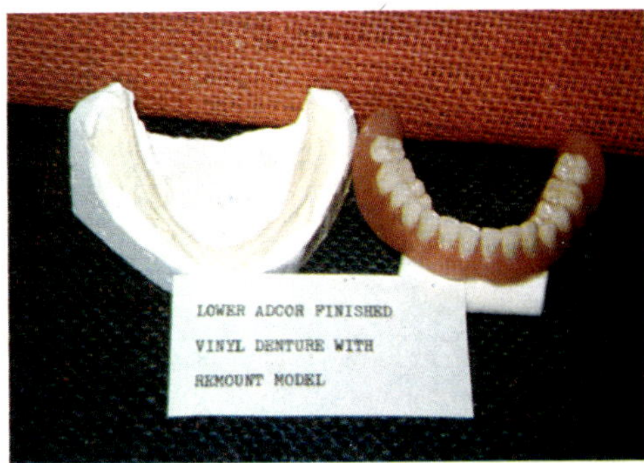

Fig. 27-7

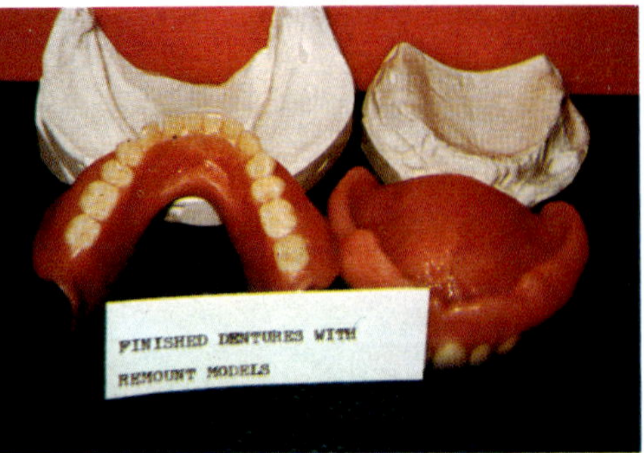

Fig. 27-8

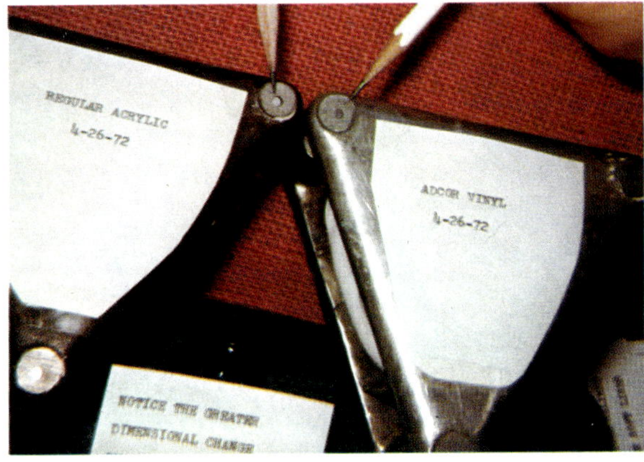

Fig. 27-9

temperature to 165° F (74° C) and cure for a minimum of 12 hours. Allow to bench cool at least 30 minutes and then cool for 20 minutes under tap water.

15. Open the flask, remove and separate the denture from the cast. Trim and polish the vinyl denture (Fig. 27-7) in the usual manner.

16. For future use prepare a remount model (cast) of the denture for checking occlusion (Fig. 27-8).

PART II

Anchored Dentures

Ajax Menekratis, D.D.S., F.I.C.D.

I dedicate this book to the late Dr. Marcel Darcissac, whose knowledge of dentistry has been a constant inspiration.

I would like to express thanks and appreciation to my very skilled technicians Claude and Gérard Goiran, whose invaluable help and patience have contributed greatly in realizing this technique; gratitude to my youngest technician Alain Pigaglio, and thanks also to my assistant Susan M. J. Nicholls, S.R.N., for her invaluable help in the planning and the writing of this book.

I also express gratitude to my friends Dr. Jack Buchman and Dr. Nathan Allen Shore who have inspired and assisted me in my work.

28. Initial Consultation

Since most of the patients coming for this type of dentistry present with mouths in a poor and often infected state, we insist that they consult their physician for a complete physical examination.

Any previous relevent medical history is considered, with particular attention to blood disorders, and cardiac and respiratory disease. Blood analysis is performed on all elderly patients and those who have been in poor health.

29. Full Mouth Radiography

Upon receiving medical clearance from the physician we proceed with the balance of our evaluation—full mouth radiography and the fabrication of study models.

It is essential that every dentist take full mouth x-rays and probe the pockets prior to the diagnostic consultation. In such cases only good radiography will reveal bone resorption in bifurcations. As I will later point out, the presence of the latter radically affects the handling of the case. Edentulous areas must also be radiographed to locate any areas of residual infection.

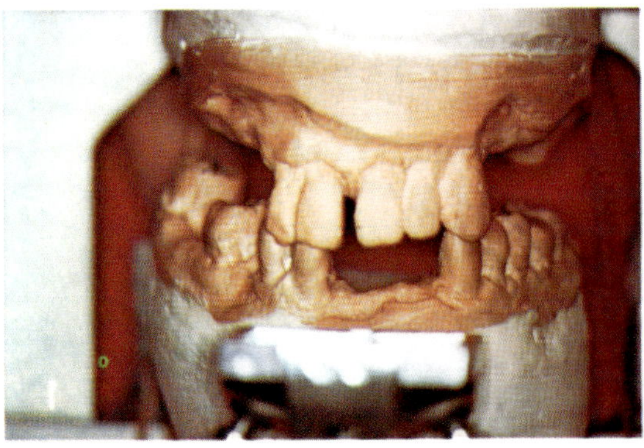

Fig. 30-1

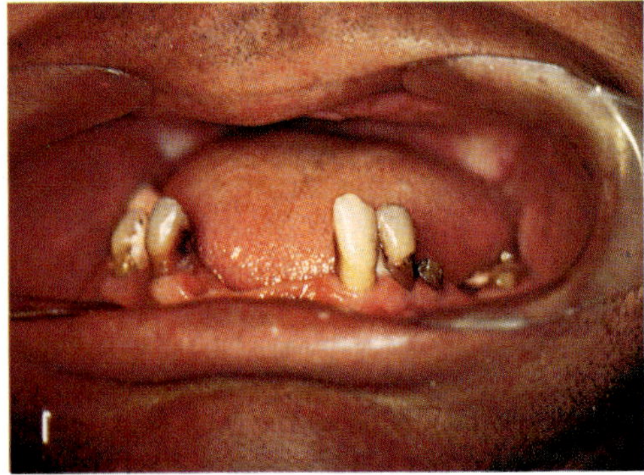

Fig. 30-2

30. Study Models

Coe alginate impressions are taken of both jaws, and plaster models prepared in the laboratory. With these in his possession the dentist has some idea of the malpositioning of the teeth and the chaotic occlusion (Fig. 30-1).

During the same session a face bow record and bite are taken using the Whip-Mix face bow. The models are mounted on the Whip-Mix articulator (Fig. 30-2).

31. Diagnostic Consultation

Here the dentist must decide which teeth are to be extracted, and at the same time review the state of those to be kept. He must also decide whether the molar roots are to be sectioned and used as individual anchors, and whether there are alveolar abnormalities such as torus palatinus, torus mandibularis or low attached frenums. Such abnormalities would interfere with the fit of the denture and, consequently, with patient comfort.

At this time also it is pointed out to the patient that at no time during treatment will he be without teeth. (Further on in this Part, I will explain how first I make partial dentures, and then, later, when the teeth are cut, full temporary dentures.)

32. Preparation of the Mouth Prior to Extractions

Before proceeding to the extraction of all the condemned teeth, a thorough scaling is necessary. Most of these patients have been negligent about dental hygiene for many years, and as a result their mouths present in a chronically infected state, with gross deposits of tartar on the teeth. It is my policy to take great care over the scaling of the teeth, even if it requires the patient's return for several sessions. At this time I always instruct in good brushing technique.

If the gums present in a poor or infected condition, it is advisable to prescribe a course of oral antibiotics with antiseptic mouthwashes. This ensures—as far as the dentist is able—that before extraction and alveolectomy the mouth has been rendered optimally clean.

(Those of my colleagues unfamiliar with alveolectomy will find guidance in any oral surgery textbook, or they can refer their patients to a specialist.)

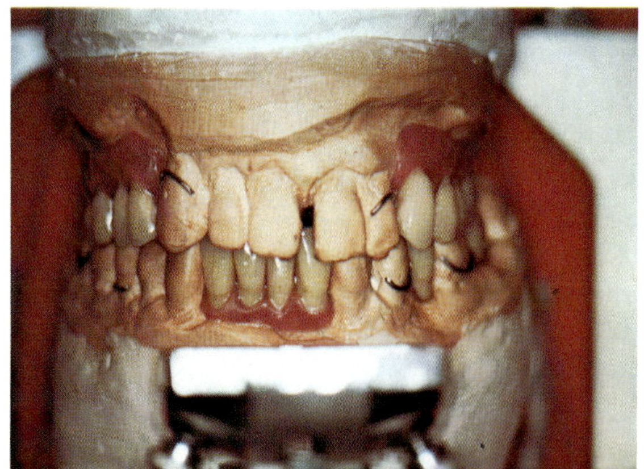
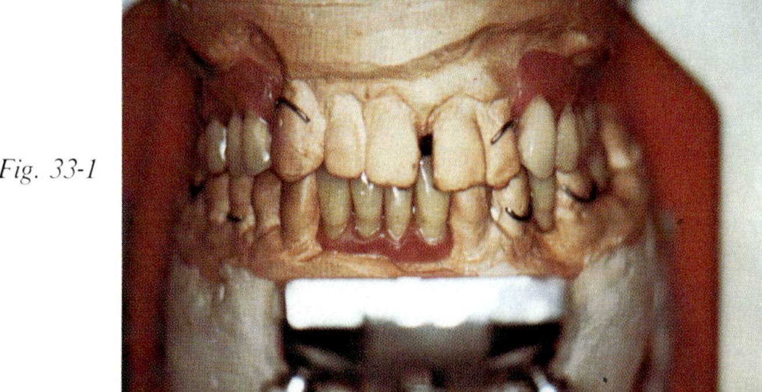

Fig. 33-1

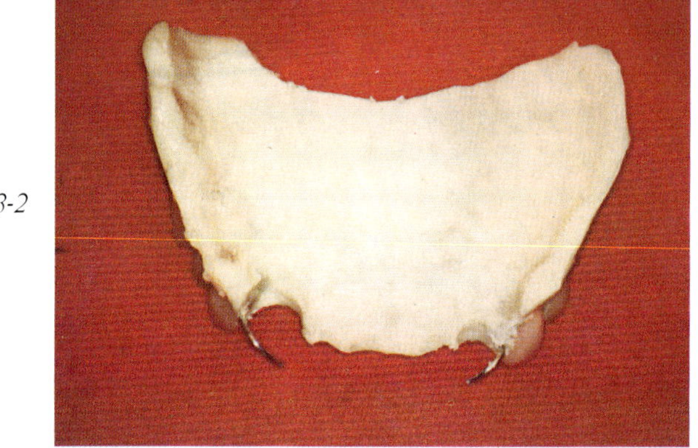

Fig. 33-2

33. Extraction and Alveolectomy

This phase can be performed under local or general anesthesia as the dentist may choose.

Using local anesthesia

The first approach is to extract the condemned teeth employing a local anesthetic. Following extraction, a Coe alginate impression is taken together with a wax bite. A temporary partial denture is made (Fig. 33-1), lined with Tic* tissue treatment material (Fig. 33-2) and placed in the mouth. The patient is sent home with instructions to return two weeks later unless problems arise earlier. The temporary partial dentures are retained by clasps, which is, however, only a temporary measure, for our next step is to perform endodontic treatment and then cut the teeth and expand the partials into full temporary anchored dentures.

Once the patient is comfortable, with the sockets clean and healing well advanced (approximately two weeks), alveolectomy is performed, if necessary, again employing a local anesthetic. The old tissue treatment is removed and the denture relined with new material. The partial denture is reinserted in the mouth over the areas that have been operated upon. The patient is sent home with instructions to return five days later for the removal of sutures. The patient now waits for complete healing—approximately two weeks.

Using general anesthesia

When extracting the condemned teeth under general anesthesia it is advisable to perform surgical procedures simultaneously. Once the patient is fully recovered from the anesthetic, Coe alginate impressions of both jaws are taken. The temporary partial dentures are prepared and fitted on tissue treatment material (TIC) as is done when employing local anesthesia, thus ensuring patient comfort. The patient is dismissed for approximately two weeks with instructions to return earlier should problems arise.

I personally recommend general anesthesia, particularly on out-of-town patients, because, not only is the number of visits reduced, but preparatory treatment of the mouth advances more rapidly. However, in the more elderly patients, and those who for one reason or another are an anesthetic risk, it is much safer to perform the work in two stages under local anesthesia, if necessary with an attending physician.

The dentist must never forget to consider each patient as an individual. All patients vary enormously in their tolerance and stamina when undergoing dental procedures. This is not only affected by age and general health: The patient's mental attitude and personality also play an enormous part. The dentist must also schedule his work to fit in with the patient's other commitments in such a way that he will be available for treatment for the period required to complete the case.

---

*This product is refined to the extent that following surgery it is well tolerated and does not decompose.

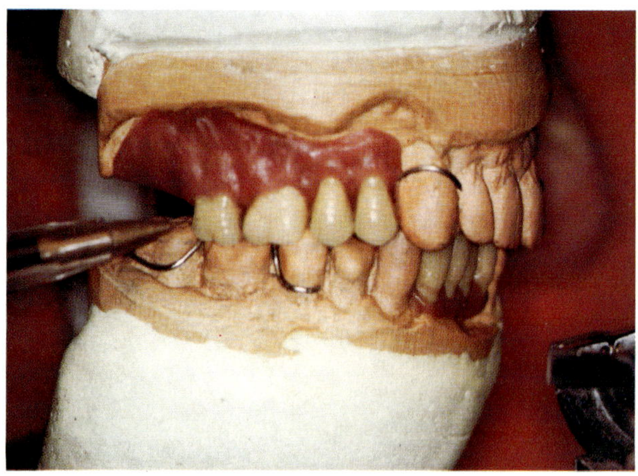

Fig. 34-1

34. Treatment of Temporomandibular Joint Dysfunction

The purpose of the previously made temporary partial dentures is to improve the aesthetics following extractions and to enable the patient to eat. In no way do they improve the occlusion of the mouth (Fig. 34-1). Usually these patients present with very poor occlusion, and the fact that they have lost teeth will in all probability have led to some degree of temporomandibular joint disturbance. Prior to treatment many of these patients have acquired bad chewing habits due to missing teeth.

To correct any temporomandibular joint disturbance we employ the technique described by Dr. Nathan Allen Shore in his book *Occlusal Equilibration and Temporomandibular Joint Dysfunction.* The use of a bite plane is inevitable. Generally speaking, it is impossible to consider the bite plane with the partial temporary dentures owing to the gross malpositioning of the teeth which exist. However, as soon as endodontic treatment has been completed and the teeth have been cut, we can build full temporary dentures with a completely flat occlusion, thus reproducing the bite plane. It is at this stage that we begin to correct the temporomandibular joint disturbances. (The technique is described in detail in Chapter 36.) No prosthetic work must ever be undertaken unless the temporomandibular joint is functioning normally.

35. Root Canal Therapy

The completed anchored denture will ultimately be fitted on pivots in roots which may be mobile as the result of considerable bone resorption. To permit the retention of pivots, these mobile teeth are cut and shaped flush with the gum. Here the dentist may be faced with either of the following eventualities: (1) the tooth may require initial devitalising and root canal therapy; (2) root canal therapy may have already been performed. If it is sound it is left *in situ,* otherwise remade. Frequently we are presented with molars that have present with bone resorption in the bifurcation. These must be endodontically treated and then cut horizontally at the line of the gum. On molars the roots are sectioned and used as individual abutments.

In regard to root canal therapy, I strongly advise the use of the rubber dam to ensure asepsis and the filling of the root canal with guttapercha cones. Whichever technique the dentist prefers when performing root canal therapy, it is of paramount importance to fill the root to the apex.

Before proceeding to further treatment, the dentist must have in his possession x-rays of all the endodontically treated teeth for future reference and verification. Much hinges on successful endodontic treatment.

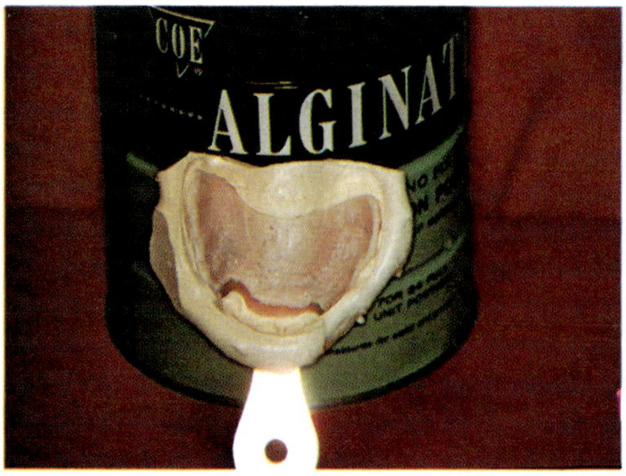

Fig. 36-1

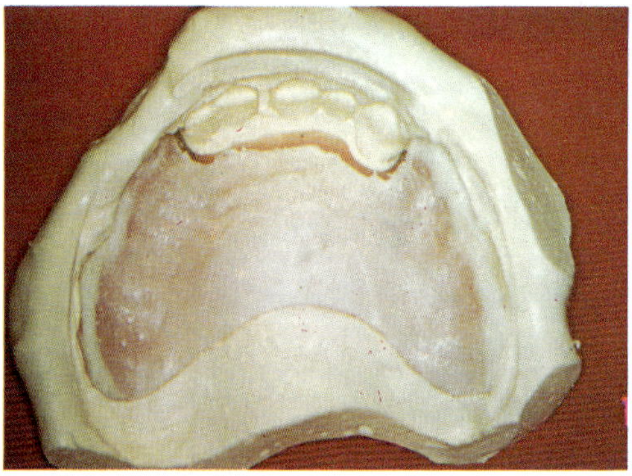

Fig. 36-2

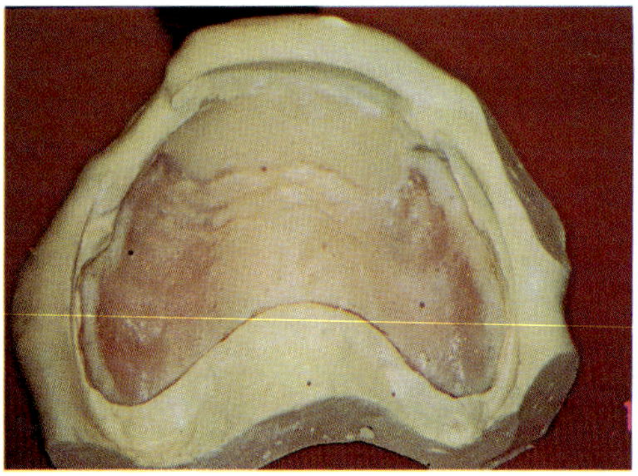

Fig. 36-3

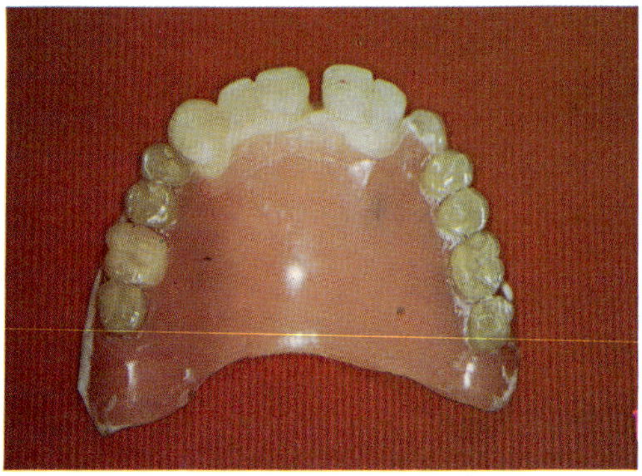

Fig. 36-4

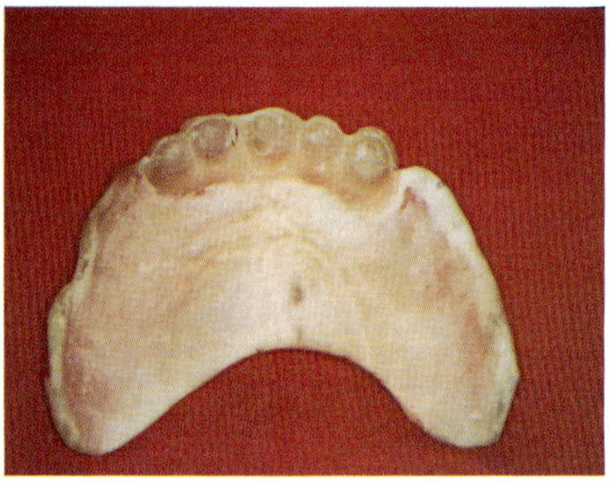

Fig. 36-5

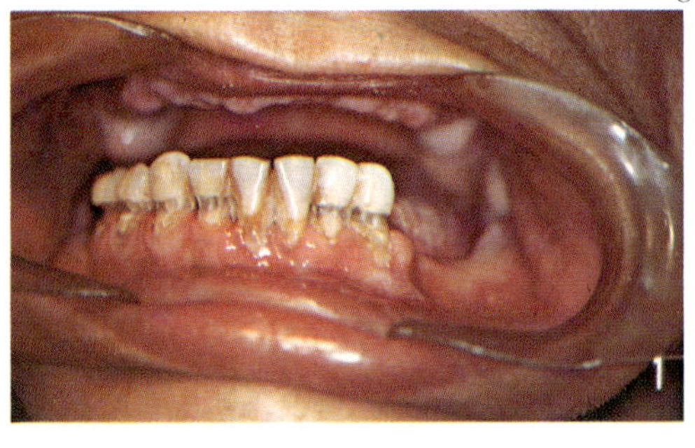

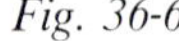

Fig. 36-6

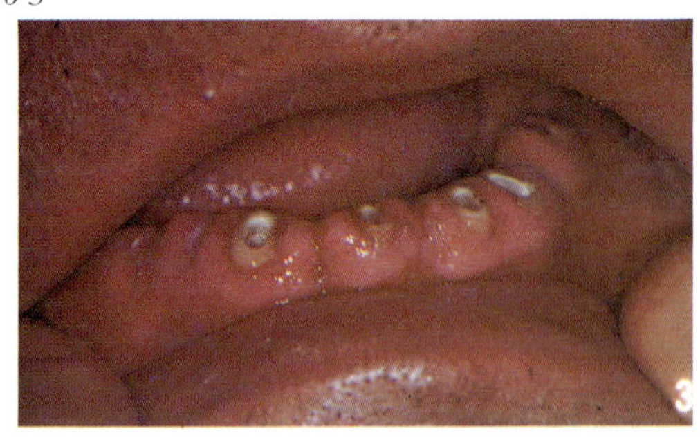

Fig. 36-7

36. Transformation of the Temporary Partial Denture to the Full Temporary Denture

At this stage the patient has a clean mouth, endodontic treatment has been completed, and a comfortable temporary partial denture lined with tissue treatment material has been constructed. We are now ready to cut the teeth and transform the temporary partial denture to the full temporary denture incorporating the endodontically treated teeth.

Alginate impressions are taken with the temporary partial denture in the mouth. Gingivectomy has not been performed at this stage. When the impression is removed the temporary partial denture is retained in the impression (Fig. 36-1). Several grooves are made (Fig. 36-2), and self-curing color-matched resin is poured in the impression and left to harden (Fig. 36-3). These new additions to the partial dentures (Fig. 36-4) are then voided, leaving only the thin outer shells which in size and shape reproduce exactly the teeth to be cut (Fig. 36-5). The teeth remaining in the mouth are now cut flush with the gum (Figs. 36-6 and 36-7).

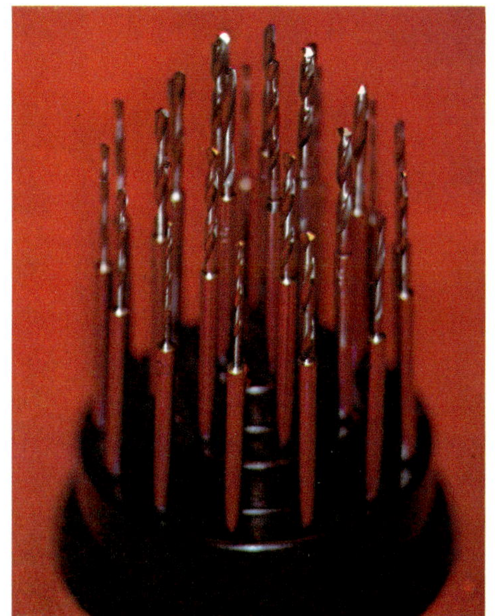

Fig. 36-8

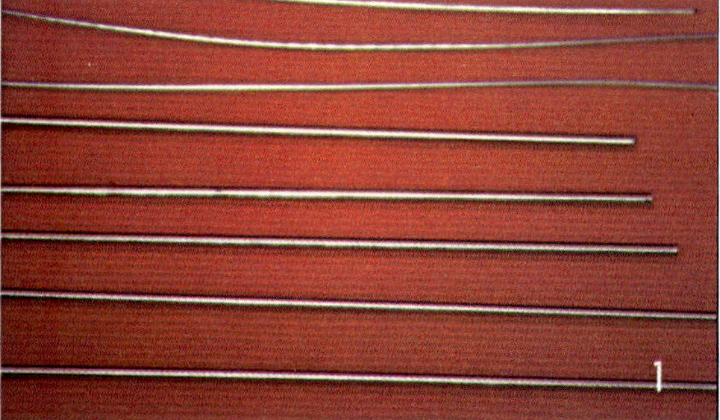

Fig. 36-9

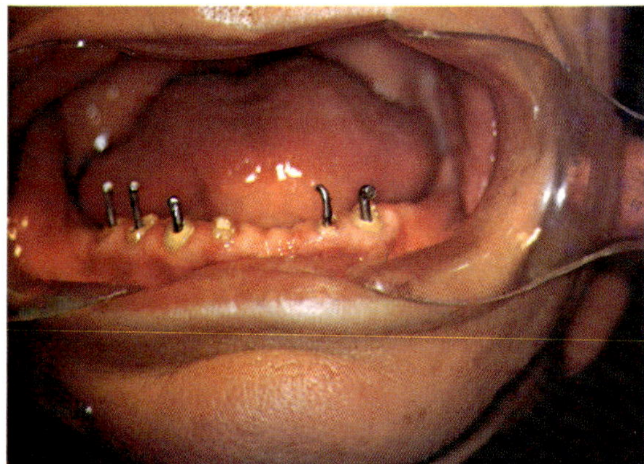

Fig. 36-10

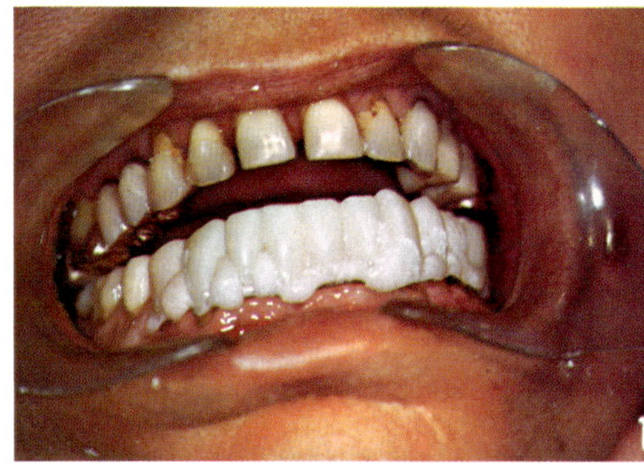

Fig. 36-11

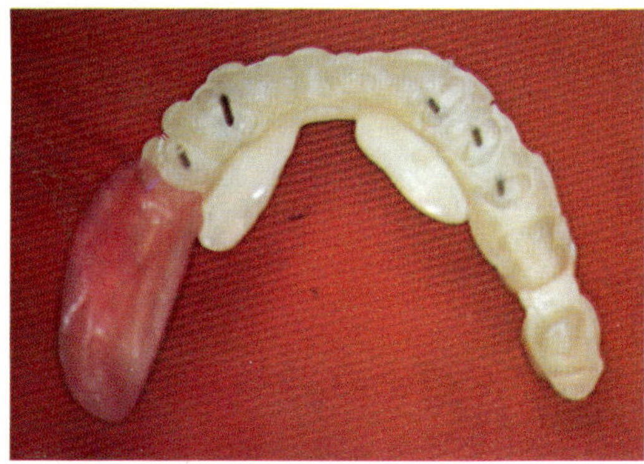

Fig. 36-12

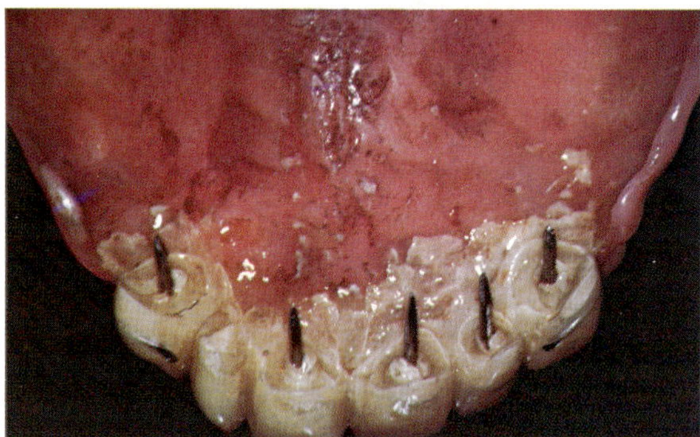

Fig. 36-13

The upper two thirds of the root canals are opened up, using calibrated Thomas drills (Fig. 36-8). Correspondingly calibrated gold/platinum alloy pivots (Fig. 36-9) are then prepared and fitted into each root (Fig. 36-10), and bent over at the top (providing a hold for the resin). Ideally the pivots must go as deep as possible into the canal, and by using similarly calibrated drills and pivots a tight fit is ensured in the canal. (Throughout this stage close radiological control is essential.)

The pivots are placed in the roots and more color-matched resin poured into the shells. The denture is then placed over the retaining pivots (Fig. 36-11). All excess resin (Fig. 36-12) is trimmed (Fig. 36-13), and the emergent complete temporary denture refitted into the mouth to ascertain patient comfort. The whole denture is then

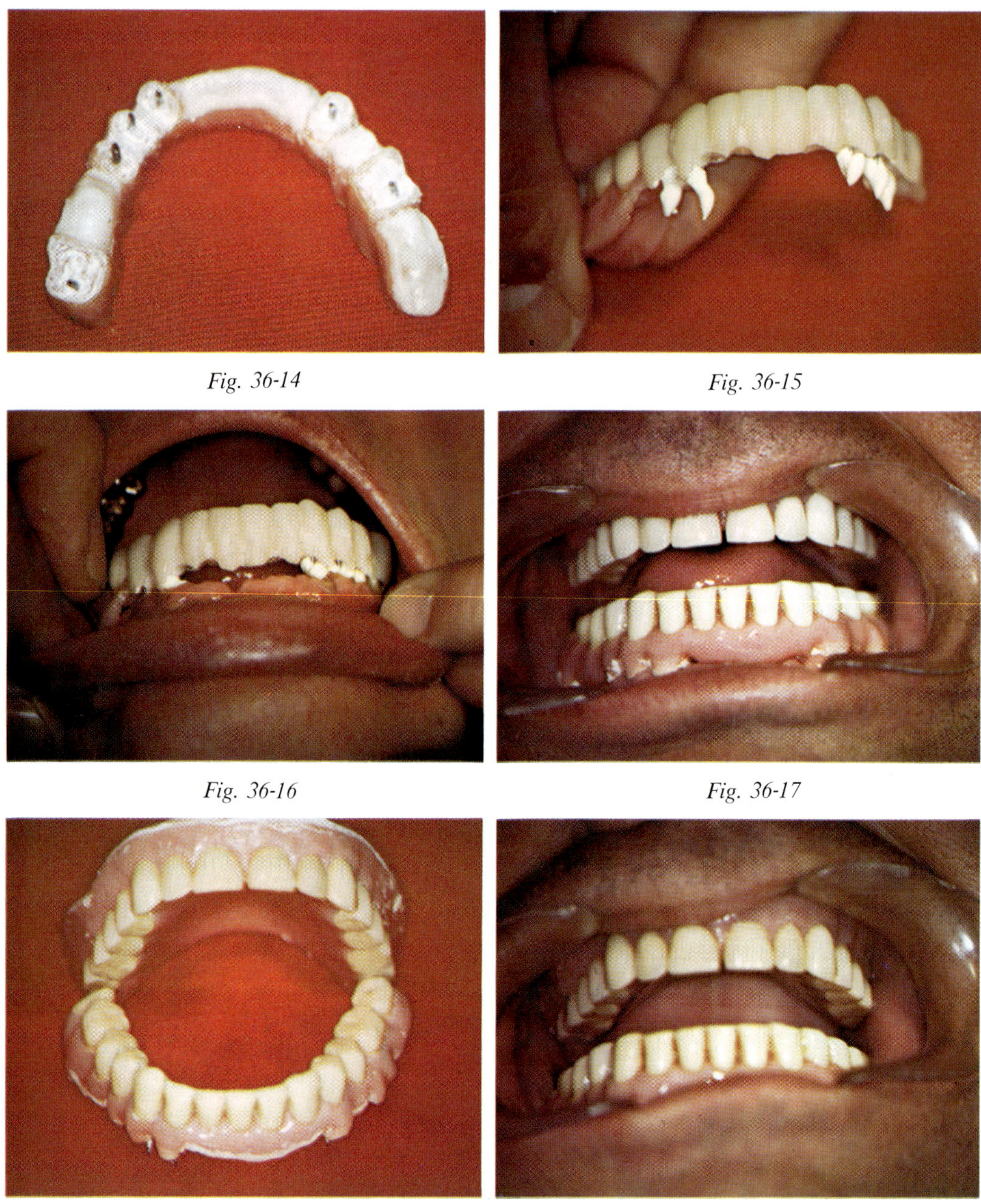

Fig. 36-14

Fig. 36-15

Fig. 36-16

Fig. 36-17

Fig. 36-18

Fig. 36-19

polished and relined with a layer of tissue treatment material (Fig. 36-14). It is then lightly cemented into position at the pivot sites with Temrex temporary cement (Figs. 36-15, 36-16 and 36-17).

At this stage occlusion must be rechecked in the mouth to ensure that it is completely flat (Fig. 36-18), thus enabling the full temporary denture to act as a bite plane (Fig. 36-19).

As the patient masticates, the mouth now automatically returns to an improved position. It is necessary to regularly adjust the occlusion, owing to the shifting of the mandible as the dysfunction of the temporomandibular joint is resolved. This is achieved by adding or subtracting acrylic on the flat occlusal surfaces of the temporary full denture. Only when this flat occlusion is achieved and the mandible is functioning normally may the dentist proceed to the next step in making anchored dentures. Malpositioning of the mandible can only result in rocking of the abutments.

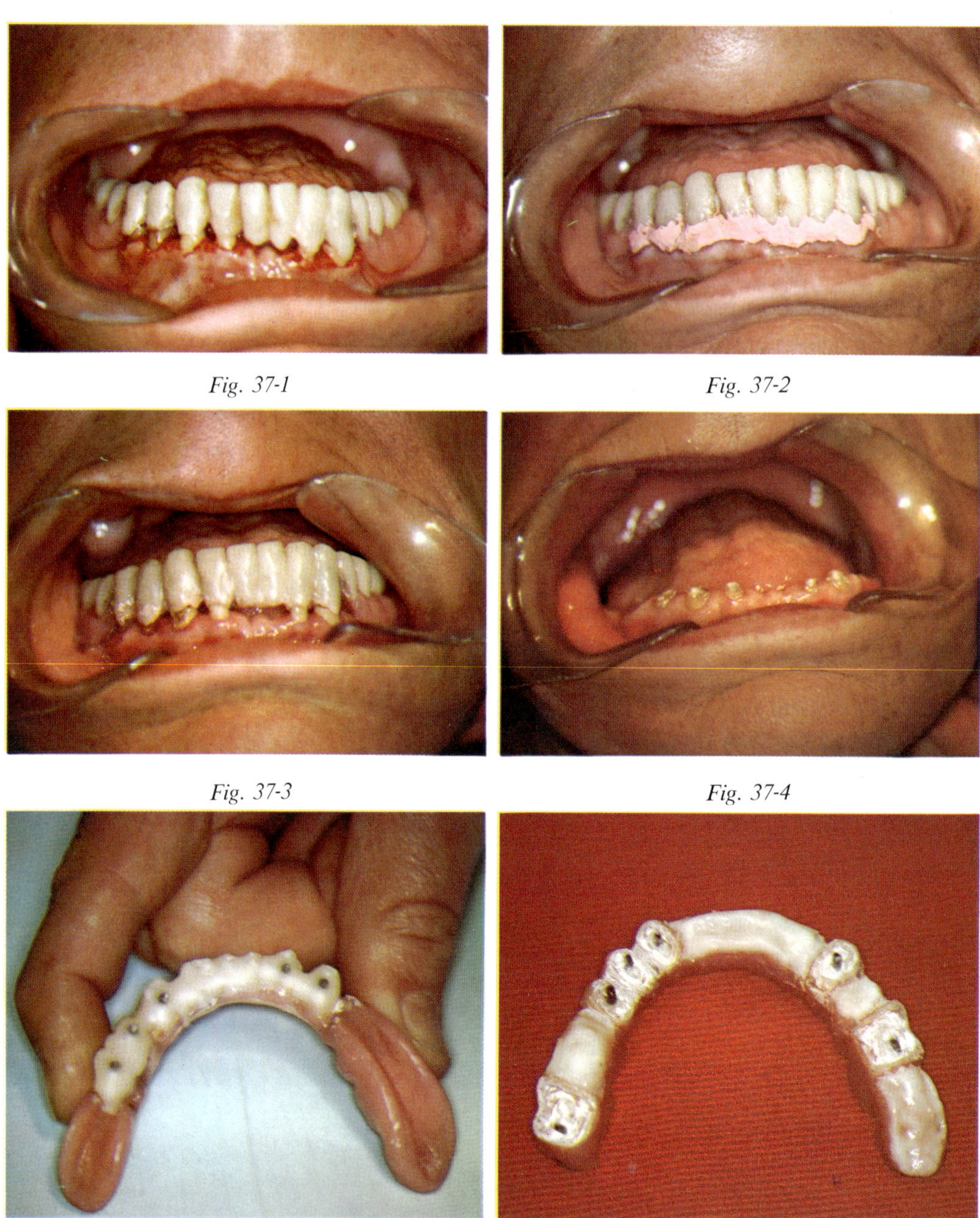

Fig. 37-1

Fig. 37-2

Fig. 37-3

Fig. 37-4

Fig. 37-5

Fig. 37-6

37. Gingivectomy

Because all these teeth present with varying degrees of periodontal involvement, I advise the radical treatment of gingivectomy. The denture is removed and the tissue treatment material scraped out. (For performing gingivectomy (Fig. 37-1) I personally recommend the use of Okun and Yudkoft knives.) Following surgery, the gums are thoroughly cleaned with saline solution. When all bleeding has stopped, the complete temporary denture is cemented in position using Ward's surgical cement (Fig. 37-2) or any other periodontal pack compound. It is usual to commence gingivectomy on the upper jaw, and the following week, if the patient is comfortable, to proceed to the lower jaw. The periodontal pack is left in position for eight days, during which period saline mouth washes are recommended to maintain oral hygiene, it being impossible to brush the teeth without disturbing the pack.

If on the eighth day following surgery the gums are not completely healed, the periodontal pack is replaced and left in position for a further eight days. When the gums are completely healed (Figs. 37-3 and 37-4), the shrinkage space between the base of the denture and the gums is filled with color-matched self-curing resin (Fig. 37-5). The complete temporary dentures are now relined with tissue treatment material (Fig. 37-6).

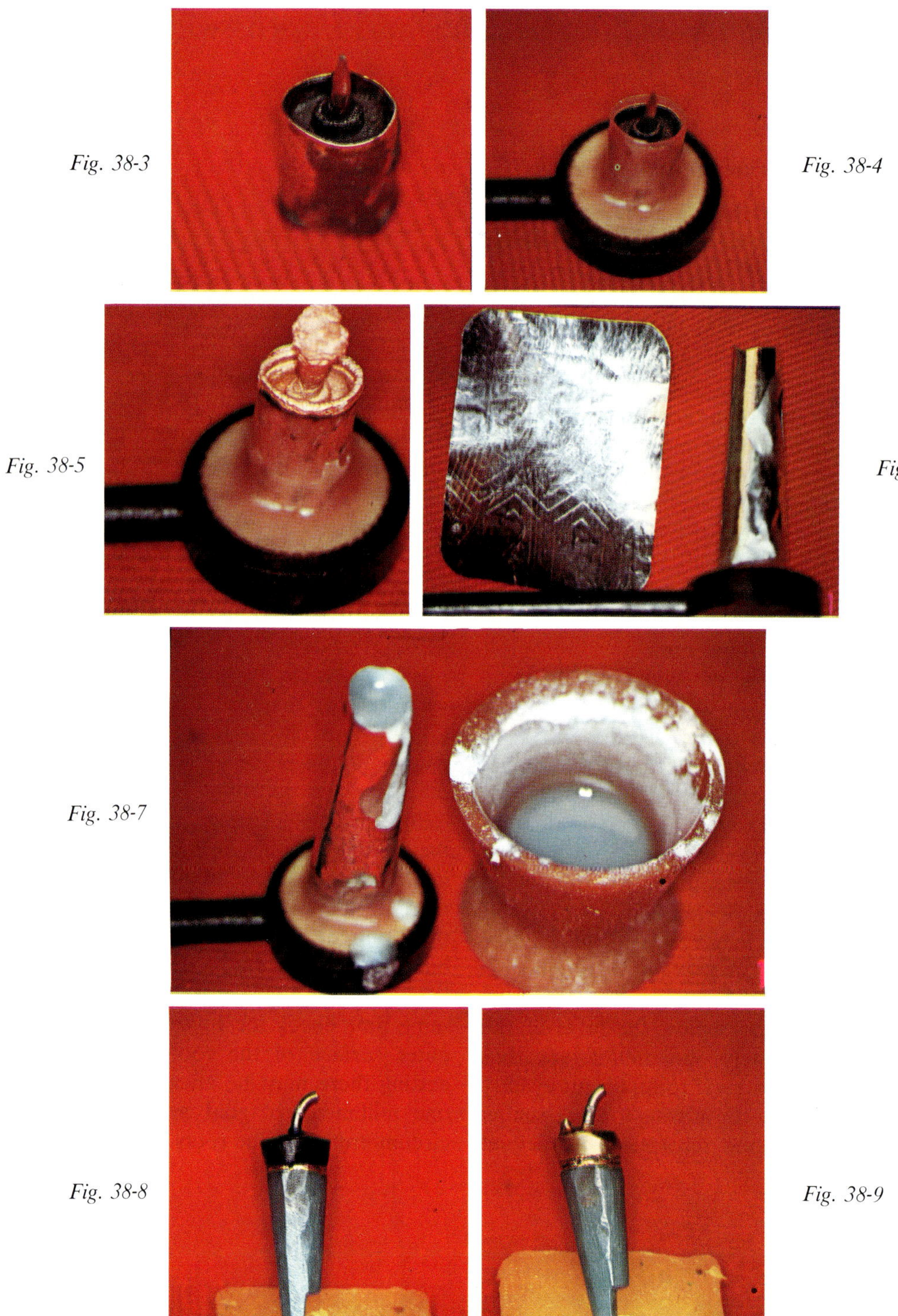

Fig. 38-3

Fig. 38-4

Fig. 38-5

Fig. 38-6

Fig. 38-7

Fig. 38-8

Fig. 38-9

The pivots are again tried in the root canals and any necessary adjustments made. X-rays are taken to ensure that the pivots fit as deeply as possible into the canal. A copper band is then adjusted, great care being exerted to ensure that the emergent part of the root is completely covered. Because the pivots have great frictional retention, which is vital to this sort of prosthetic work, it is impossible to employ hydrocolloids or silicones when taking the impressions. I have therefore, after much trial and error, concluded that the safest and most accurate form of impression involves copper bands and the use of Kerr's green stick compound.

After the copper bands have been taken (Fig. 38-3), each band is placed in an individual envelope, clearly marked with the patient's name and the number of the tooth, thus greatly facilitating work in the laboratory. Before placing the copper band impression with the pivot *in situ* into the copper plating unit it is necessary to place a small amount of wax around the outside of the pivot (Fig. 38-4). This greatly facilitates its removal from the copper plated die. The tubes are then copper plated using a Hanau electroforming unit, thus rendering copper plated dies with a pivot inside (Fig. 38-5). The copper plated die is wrapped with tin foil (Fig. 38-6), and self-curing resin is poured to build a pivot under the die (Fig. 38-7). On completion of the plating, the technician waxes up the die with the pivot in place in order to cast a gold transfer (Fig. 38-8). These transfers are cast in 22-karat gold (Fig. 38-9). The transfers are then fitted onto the prepared abutments, and a final check is made to fit

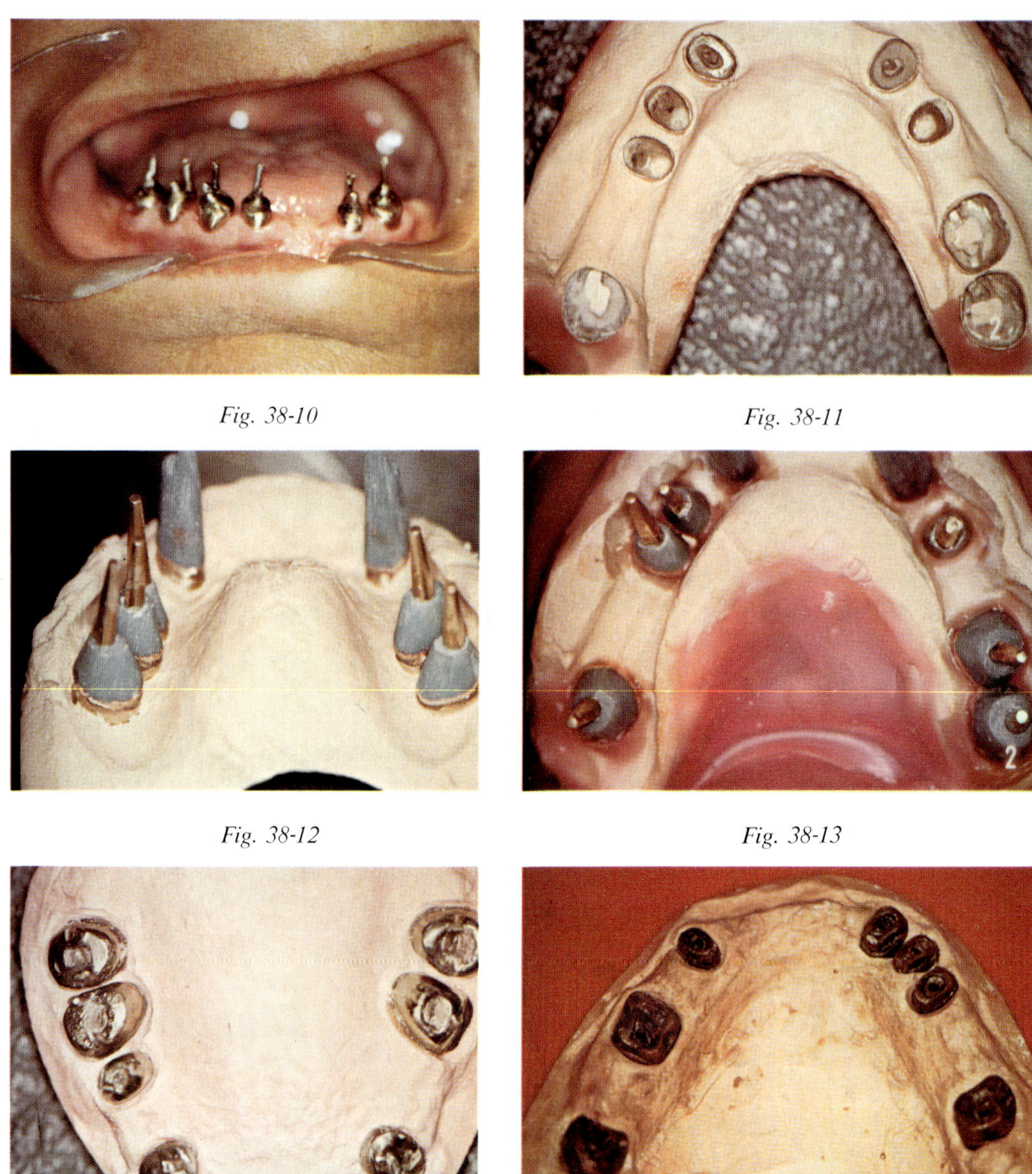

Fig. 38-10

Fig. 38-11

Fig. 38-12

Fig. 38-13

Fig. 38-14

Fig. 38-15

and complete coverage of the root (Fig. 38-10). If there is any discrepancy the tube-impression is retaken and another transfer prepared. Once all the transfers are satisfactory they are fitted in the mouth and full plaster impressions taken (Fig. 38-11). Dies are positioned into gold transfers (Fig. 38-12). These impressions are then boxed and poured in a hard stone composition (Fig. 38-13). The model (Fig. 38-14) is now trimmed and the transfers removed (Fig. 38-15).

The patient is now wearing full temporary dentures retained by pivots, with tissue treatment material on the inner surface. Since this temporary denture is cemented in the patient's mouth with temporary cement (Temrex), it is a simple task for the dentist to remove the denture and clean it as necessary.

I cannot stress enough the importance of a bite plane which functions on a flat occlusion, thus attaining optimal normal mandibular function. The proof for the dentist that normal mandibular function is being achieved is the observation that the mobility of the roots is diminishing and the temporomandibular joint is functioning normally.

Anchored dentures is the name I have given to this type of prosthesis. Upon consultation, these patients would in the past have been diagnosed as candidates for full dentures. I have found, however, that solidly implanted roots can, whatever their length, and providing all the intermediate treatment has been conscientiously carried out, be used as an anchor.

We are now in possession of two plaster models with copper-plated abutments. The dentist is now confronted with three possible contingencies:

1. Teeth remaining in both the upper and lower jaws.

2. Teeth in the lower jaw but not in the upper.

3. Teeth in the upper jaw but not in the lower (which is rarely seen).

Whichever variation presents to the dentist both upper and lower jaws are treated alike. From this point onwards I shall consider that the patient is edentulous despite the fact that we have abutments in position.

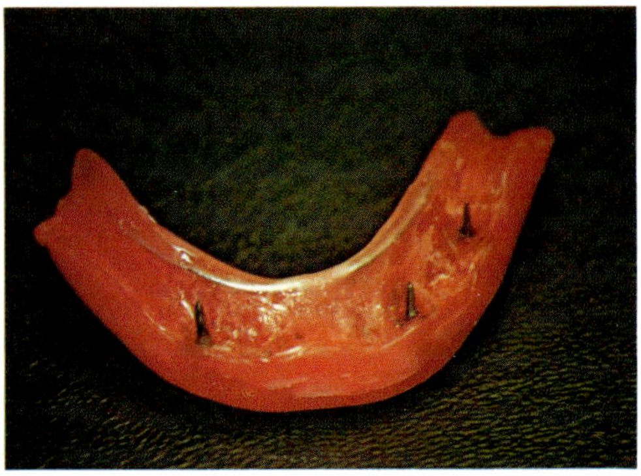

Fig. 39-1

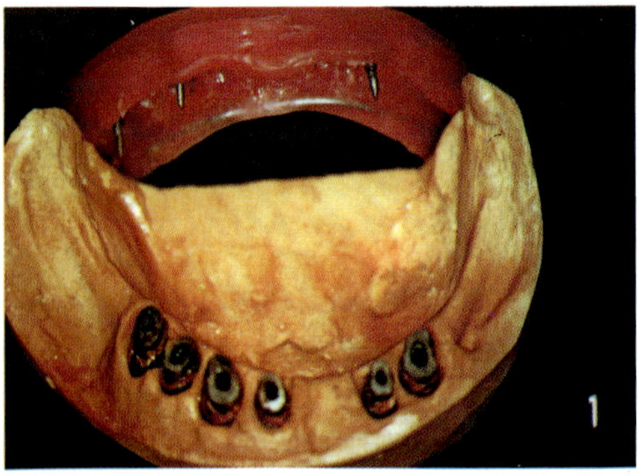

Fig. 39-2

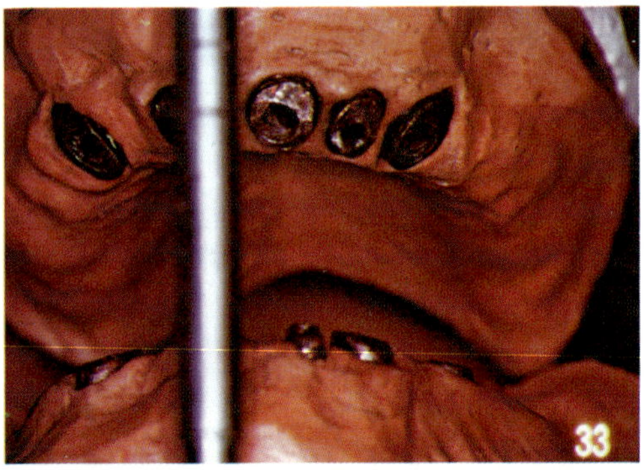

Fig. 39-3

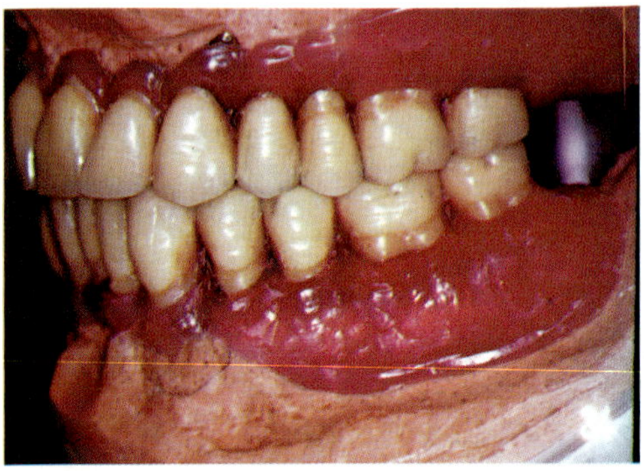

Fig. 39-4

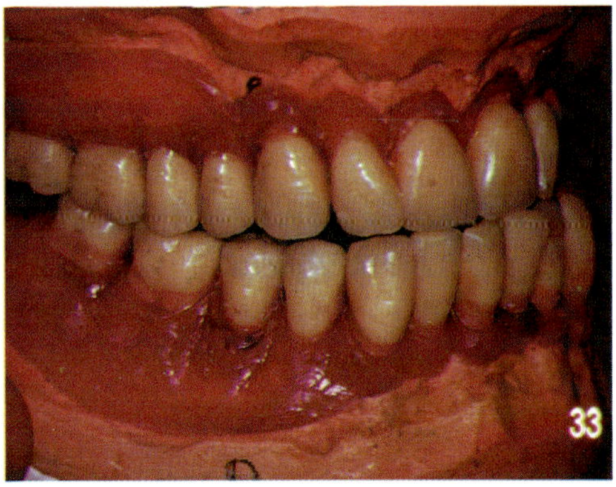

Fig. 39-5

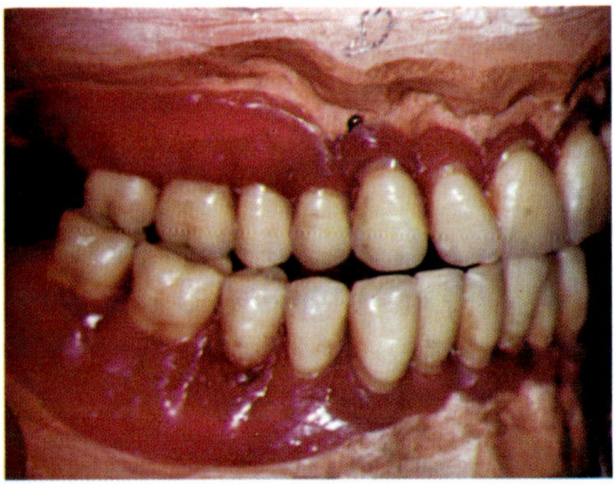

Fig. 39-6

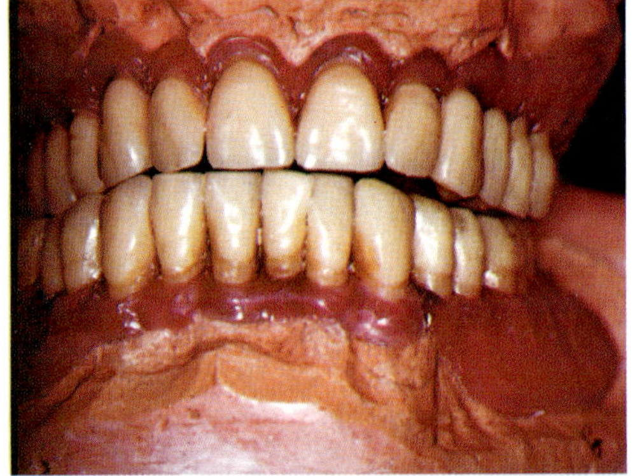

Fig. 39-7

39. Full Wax Denture

Our next task is to produce full dentures in wax (employing the Buchman technique described in Part I). In order to stabilise the wax bite blocks it is advisable to place two or three root canal pivots into the prepared roots (Fig. 39-1). Over these pivots (Fig. 39-2), bite blocks are built using the Buchman procedure as described in Chapter 4. After the bite blocks have been made, follow the procedure for the taking of vertical and centric dimension (Chapter 9), the mounting of these bite blocks on the Whip-Mix articulator, and the setting up of the teeth. Now in possession of full wax dentures, we can set them on the Whip-Mix articulator. At this stage (Figs. 39-3 to 39-7) the position of the roots does not necessarily correspond with the teeth set in the wax denture. The positioning is unimportant however, for we still regard the patient as having no roots.

We must never forget that in these cases patients present with a history of missing teeth, thus resulting in gross displacement of some or all of the remaining teeth. The form of displacement may present as diastema, migration, rotation, tilting and so on. However, in the particular case that I am going to discuss, we have a substantial layer of pink wax covering the gums over the roots, due to excessive bone resorption.

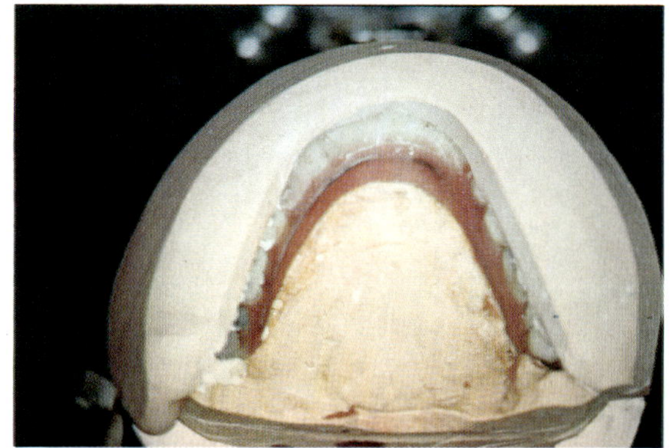

Fig. 39-8

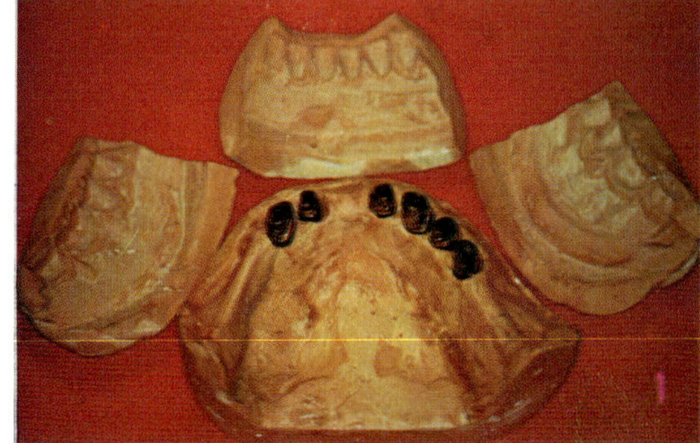

Fig. 39-9

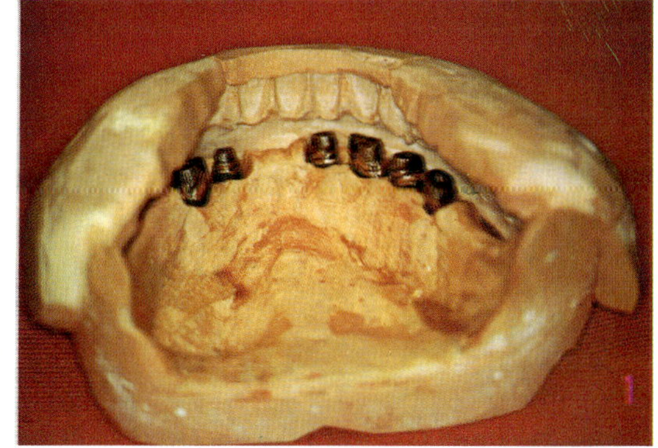

Fig. 39-10

The wax dentures are fitted in the mouth, and if the occlusion and vertical dimension are correct, we begin to construct the regular anchored denture. The first step is to make plaster cores to fix the final position of the teeth (Fig. 39-8). The cores are prepared in stone in three sections:

1. The left molars and bicuspids.
2. The right molars and bicuspids.
3. The incisors.

These together form an interlocking unit. This is achieved by forming (1) and (2) simultaneously, and then fitting the final segment (3).

When the plaster cores have hardened, the wax is boiled out (Fig. 39-9) and the cores are remounted on the model, thus giving accurate positioning of the teeth (Fig. 39-10).

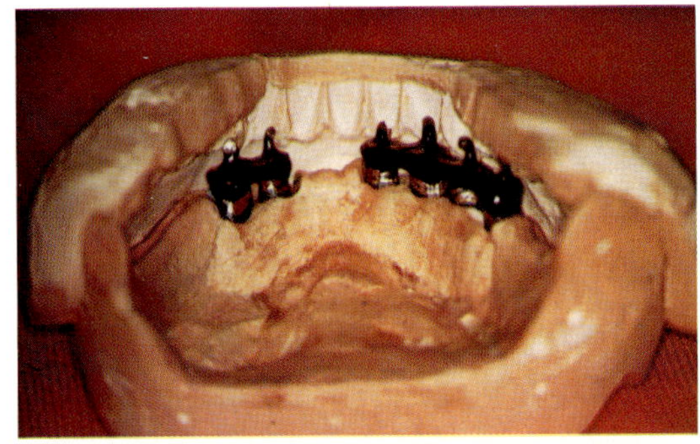
Fig. 40-1

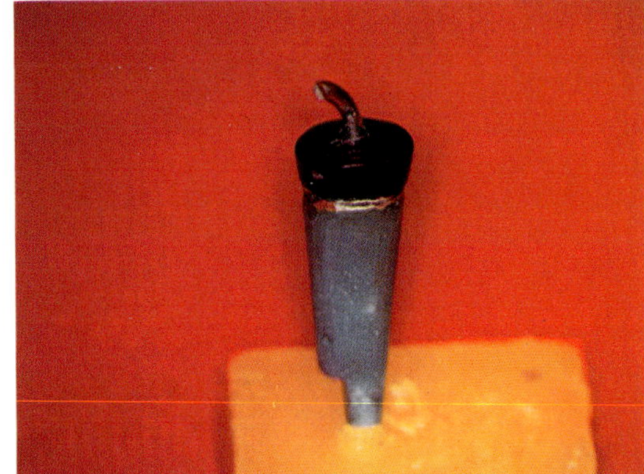
Fig. 40-2

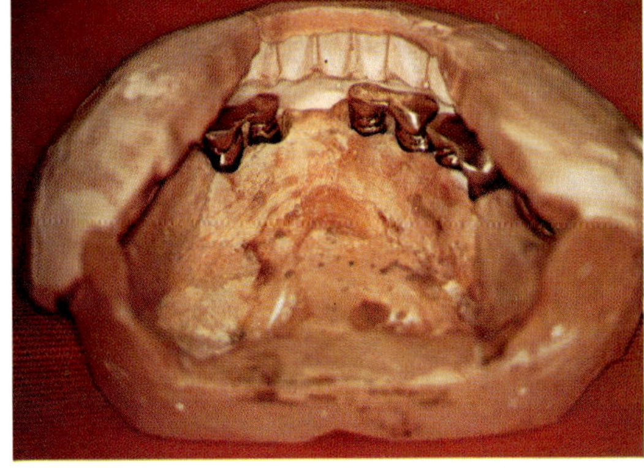
Fig. 40-3

40. Attachments

It is only now that the full impact of the malpositioning of the teeth may be realised. For all roots we build gold caps, which in turn support the precision attachments. Blue inlay wax (Fig. 40-1) is used for this procedure. The lower part of the waxing that circumscribes the root must project upwards in a funnel-shaped fashion (Fig. 40-2), thus preventing new gum growth covering the roots and ultimately destroying the fit. At the apex a reversed funnel shape is used. (I have frequently observed new gum growth in classical bridge work, due to the fact that oral anatomy was not respected during the shaping of the teeth.) The occlusal surface of the gold caps on which the precision attachments will be soldered must be absolutely flat (Fig. 40-3). To achieve precision work at this stage I employ a parallelometer. For all the metal frames and castings I use gold and its special solder. I use both ready- and custom-made attachments.

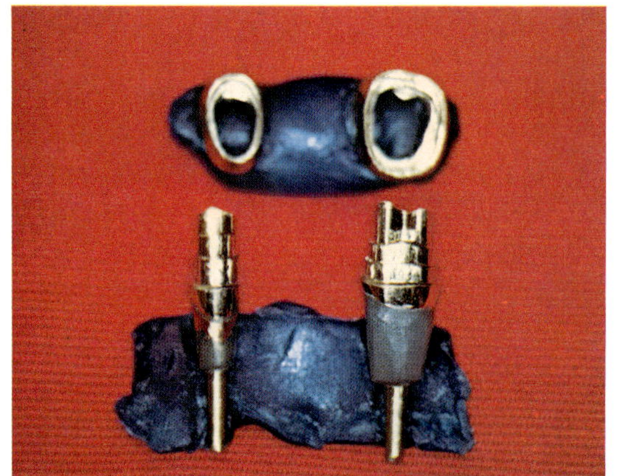

Fig. 40-4

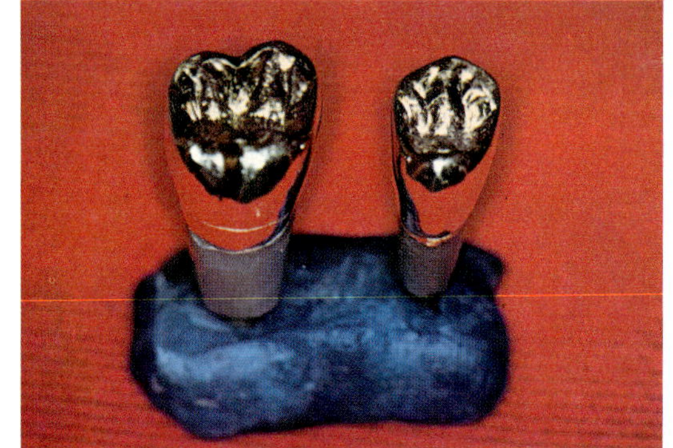

Fig. 40-5

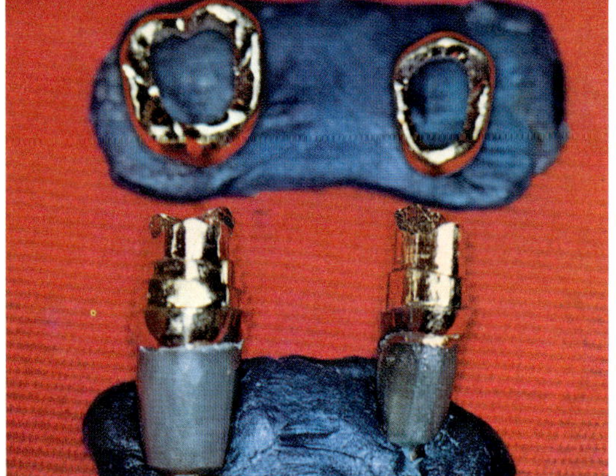

Fig. 40-6

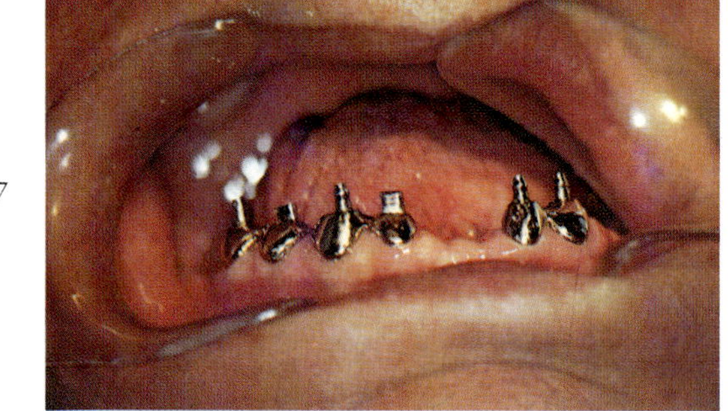

Fig. 40-7

Ready made attachments. Although there are a great variety of ready made attachments available, I have used the following personally:

1. Gerber N° 686.
2. Gerber N° 686 a.
3. Dolla Bona N° 604.
4. Gerber hinge N° 716 a.

These are all supplied with fixation bars.

Custom made attachments. These I make myself in the laboratory. They include: (1) telescopic crowns (Figs. 40-4, 40-5 and 40-6), (2) gold squares, which I solder onto the root when there is no necessity to fit a precision attachment, preventing rotation of the denture (Fig. 40-7). I believe that the attachments I make myself are invariably the most simple, and after 14 years' experience, I seen no reason to substitute more complex techniques. As the Gerber is the most frequently used attachment, we should review its use.

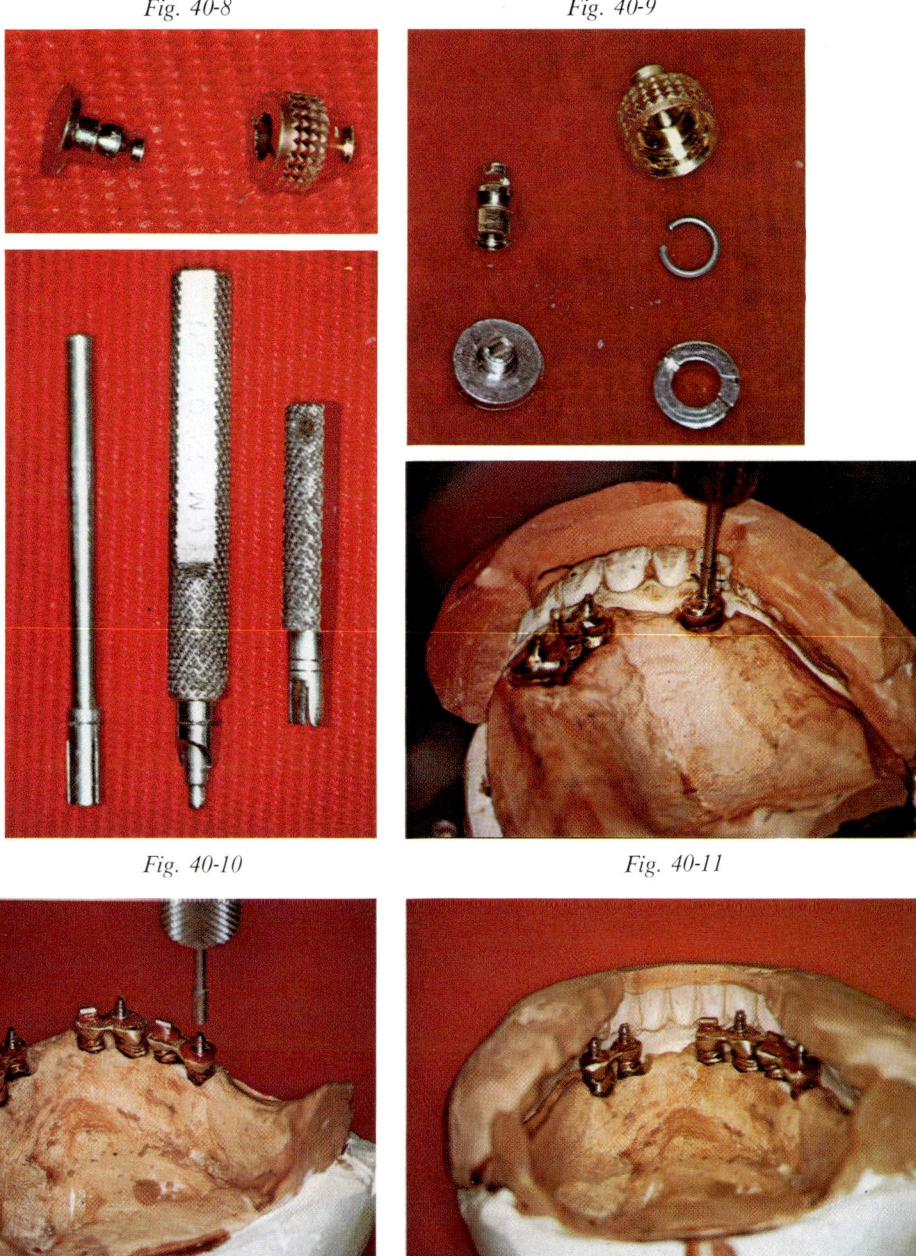

Fig. 40-8

Fig. 40-9

Fig. 40-10

Fig. 40-11

Fig. 40-12

Fig. 40-13

1. Gerber attachment (Figs. 40-8 and 40-9).
2. Gerber sticks (Fig. 40-10).
3. Gerber attachment mounted on the parallelometer (Fig. 40-11).
4. Positioning the Gerber (Fig 40-12).
5. Waxing the Gerber (Fig. 40-13).
6. Soldering the Gerber: as for any attachment.

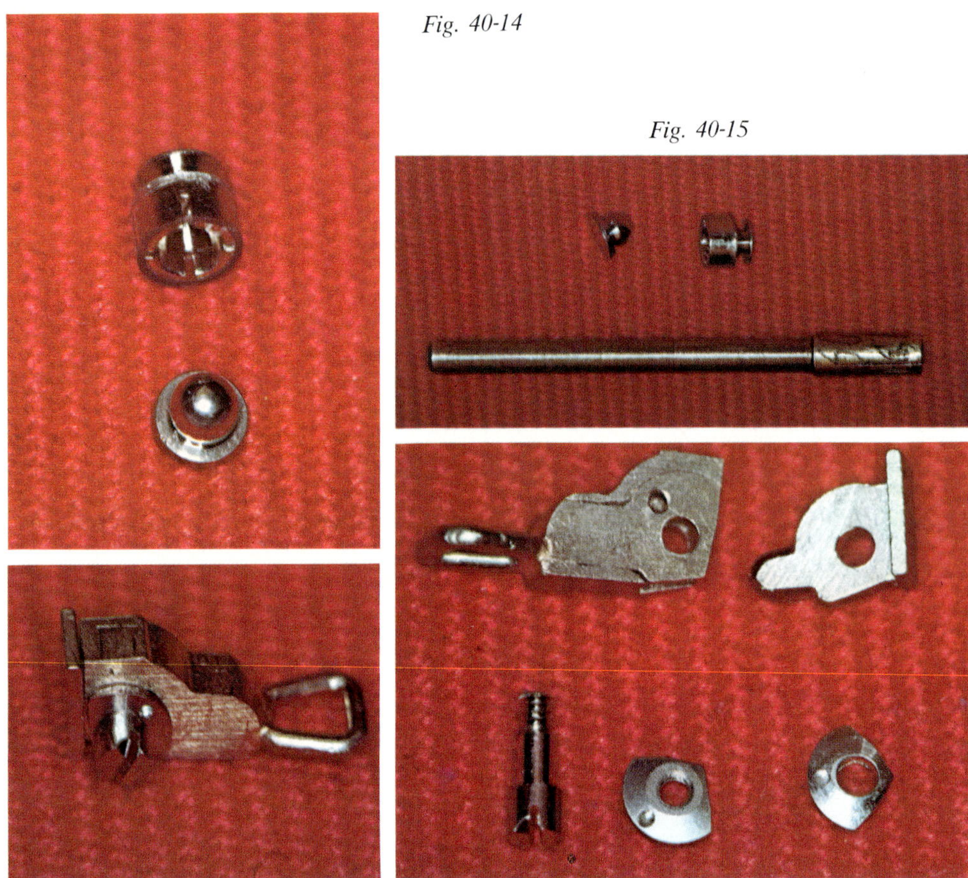

Fig. 40-14

Fig. 40-15

Fig. 40-16

Fig. 40-17

The Dolla Bona (Figs. 40-14 and 40-15). The Dolla Bona is fitted in exactly the same way as the Gerber. It is however only employed if there is insufficient vertical height. Unfortunately though, with less height there is diminished frictional retention.

The Gerber hinge (Figs. 40-16 and 40-17). A hinge is never used on the upper jaw, because the palatal bar prevents rocking of the denture in an anterior posterior direction. Regarding the lower jaw, we always use a hinge for free-end saddles replacing bicuspids and molars. If the hinge is not present, we are fostering the destruction of the anterior abutment. If any recession should occur under the free-end saddle over a period of time, it is a simple procedure, if the hinge is used, to rebase the under surface of the saddle and restore good occlusal contact.

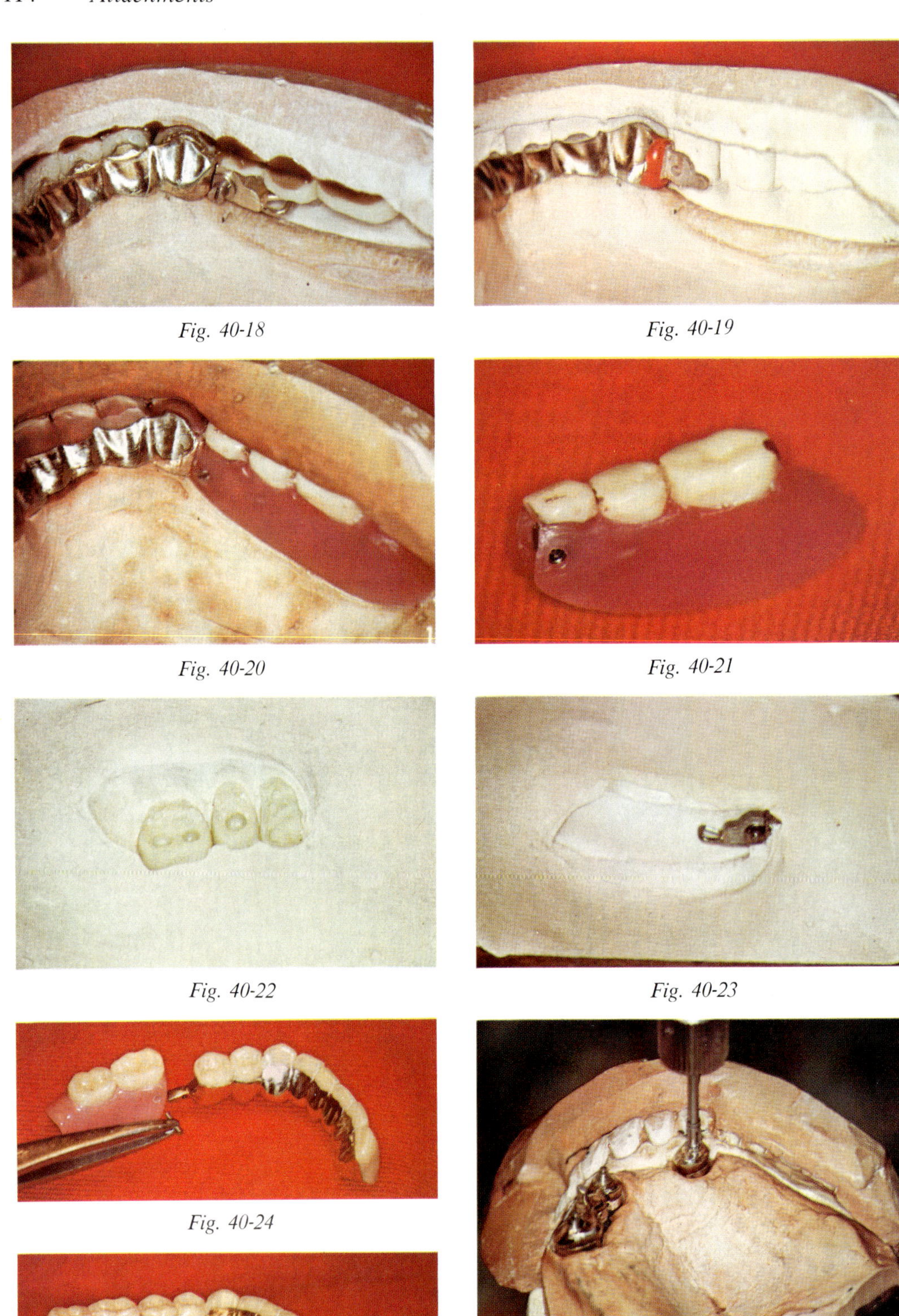

Fig. 40-18

Fig. 40-19

Fig. 40-20

Fig. 40-21

Fig. 40-22

Fig. 40-23

Fig. 40-24

Fig. 40-26

Fig. 40-25

Technique for fixing the Gerber hinge

As we have shown previously, plaster cores are made to locate the position of the teeth. The teeth over the hinge are then ground to make sufficient space for the hinge to be inserted (Fig. 40-18). At this stage we fix the male part of the hinge with sticking wax onto the frame (Fig. 40-19), and then solder this part to the frame. We now reposition the frame with the soldered hinge on the model, reposition the facings in the cores, and fix the facings to the frame with pink wax (Fig. 40-20). When the plaster cores are removed we are now in possession of the teeth held with pink wax retaining the female part of the hinge (Fig. 40-21). The saddle is now flasked as for a complete denture (Chapter 41). Thus the teeth are retained in one half of the flask and the female part of the hinge in the other. The wax is boiled out; we have in one part the facings grooved for retention (Fig. 40-23), and in the other the female part of the hinge (Fig. 40-22). The introduction of pink Huelon resin is the same as for a full denture (Chapter 41). The free end saddle is now deflasked, sandpapered and polished, and attached to the male part of the hinge by means of a transverse screw (Figs. 40-24 and 40-25). It is not necessary to fit custom or ready made attachments to all the roots. If some of the roots are weak but will provide a rest, we build gold squares on top of the root.

We now continue with the technique for building the frame of the anchored denture with its attachments. Once all the male attachments have been soldered to the gold cups, the model is remounted on the parallelometer and the position of the male attachments verified (Fig. 40-26). This is a vital control: if any discrepancies are found, the male parts must be repositioned and resoldered. We refit the plaster cores on the model to make a final check, thus ensuring that the attachments have been soldered in the correct position.

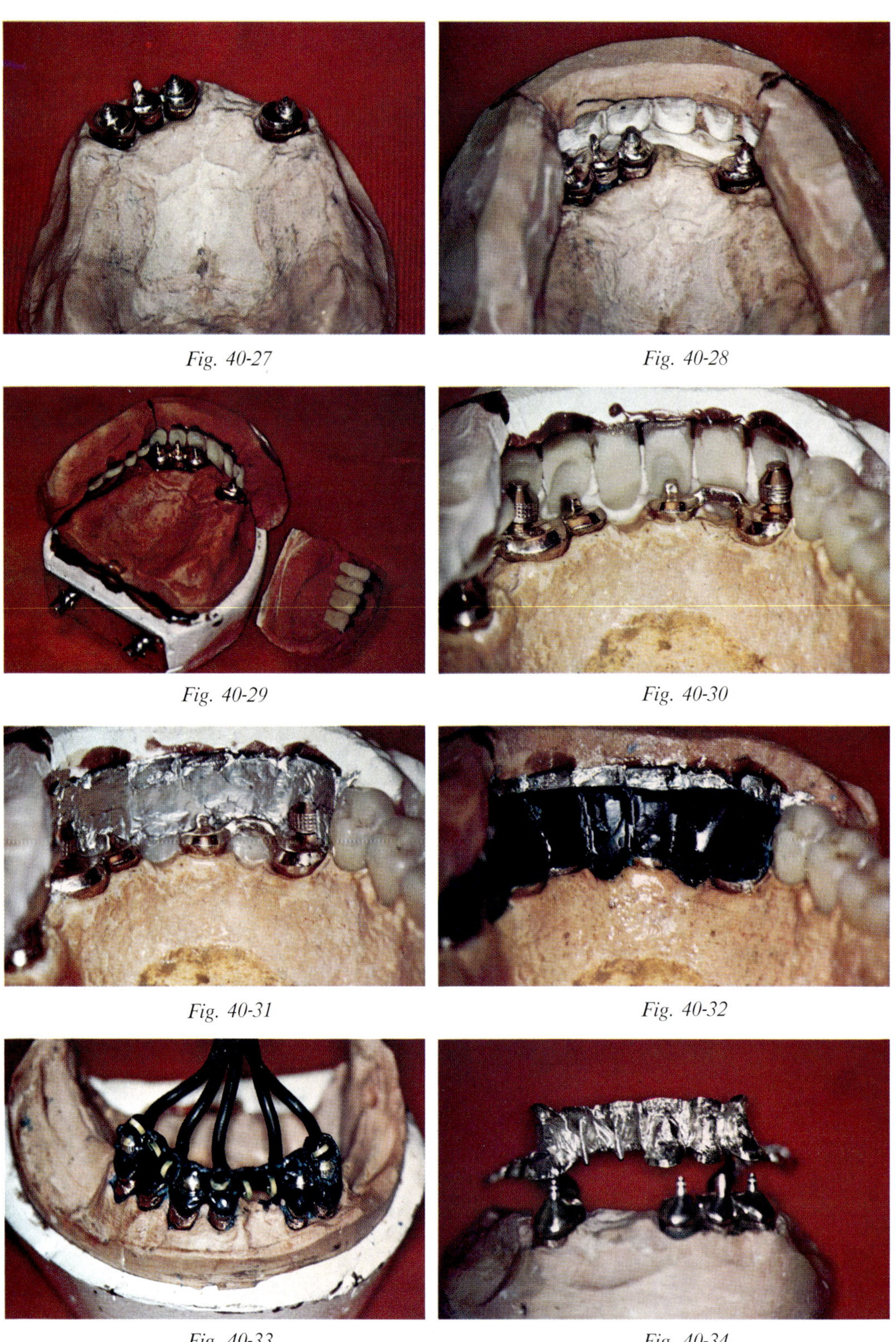

Fig. 40-27

Fig. 40-28

Fig. 40-29

Fig. 40-30

Fig. 40-31

Fig. 40-32

Fig. 40-33

Fig. 40-34

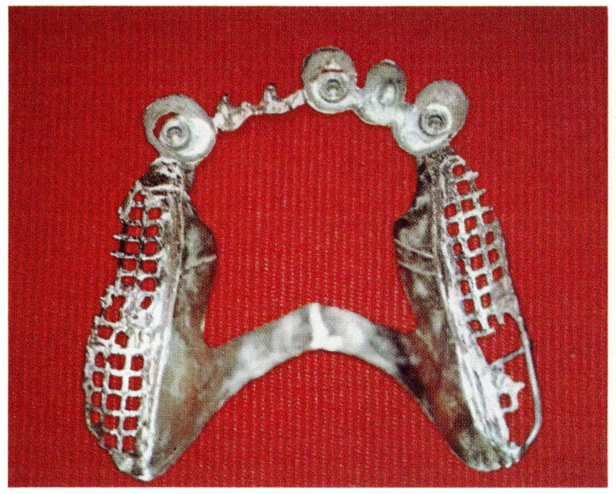

Fig. 40-35

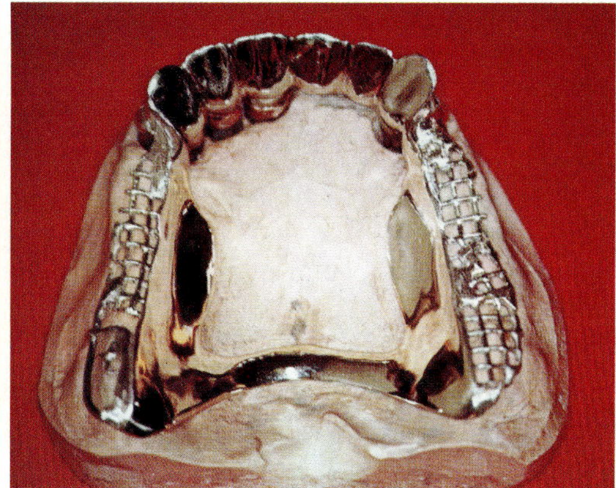

Fig. 40-36

We are now in possession of a model with all the male attachments soldered (Fig. 40-27). The next step is to introduce the female attachments onto the males (Fig. 40-28). The plaster cores are now repositioned supporting the teeth, and we grind all the teeth opposite the attachments into facings (Figs. 40-29 and 40-30). We can now see how much space exists between the facings and the female attachments. If it is insufficient the facings are ground down further. Tin foil (Fig. 40-31) is applied on the inner surface of the facings. We pour blue wax onto the tin foil and over the attachments and caps (Fig. 40-32). The sprued wax form (Fig. 40-33) will represent the metal frame. The anterior wax frame is invested and cast, and the female attachments soldered on (Fig. 40-34). The upper palatal frame is waxed, and the cast soldered to the anterior portion (Fig. 40-35). We now fit the frame with its soldered female attachments onto the model (Fig. 40-36). At this stage there must be no rocking, which may be caused by: (1) the female attachments being malpositioned owing to inaccurate soldering, or (2) the custom made attachments not being parallel to the ready made attachments which have already been soldered. If all is satisfactory we proceed to the next step.

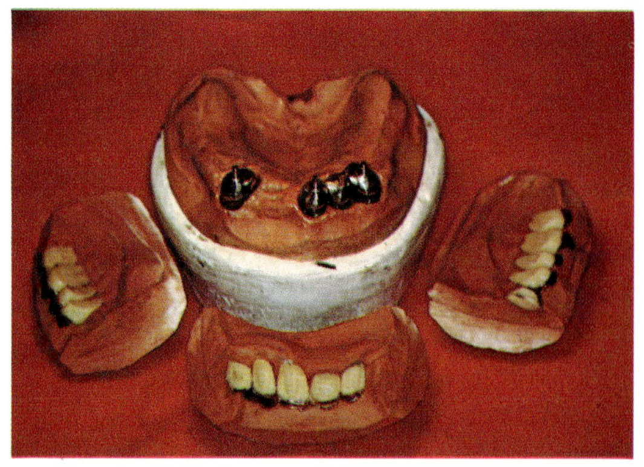

Fig. 40-37

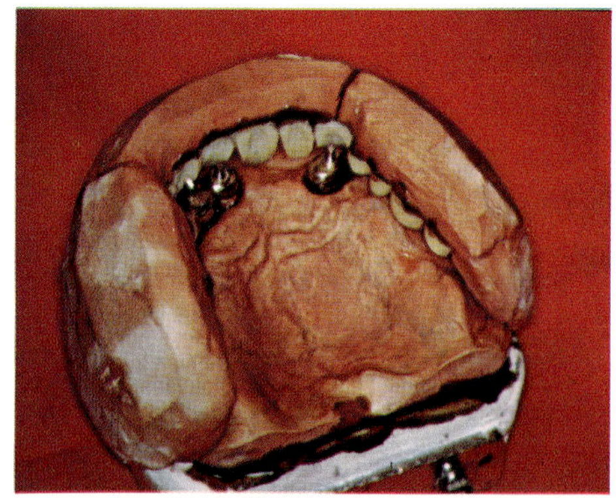

Fig. 40-38

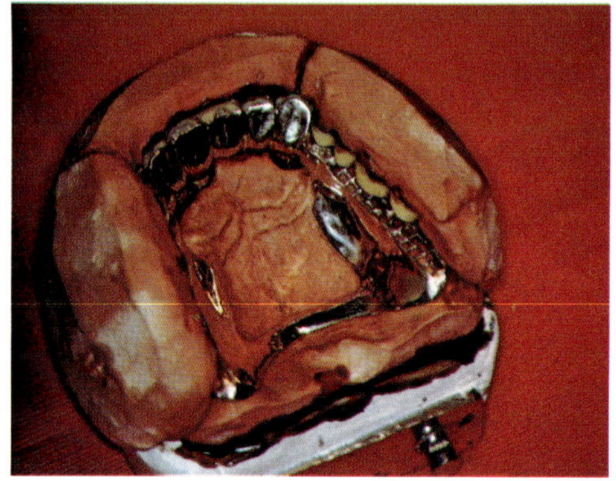

Fig. 40-39

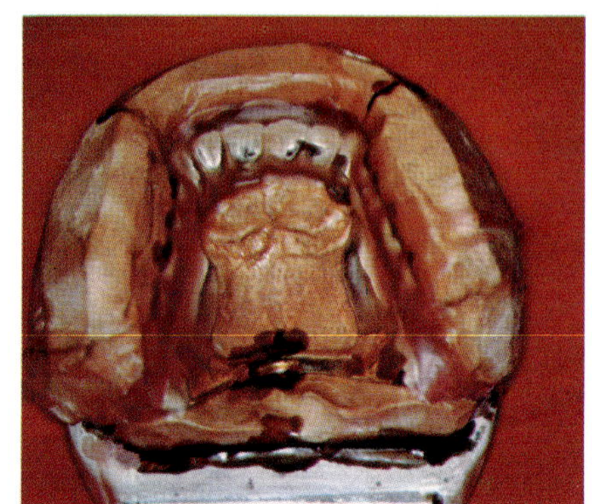

Fig. 40-40

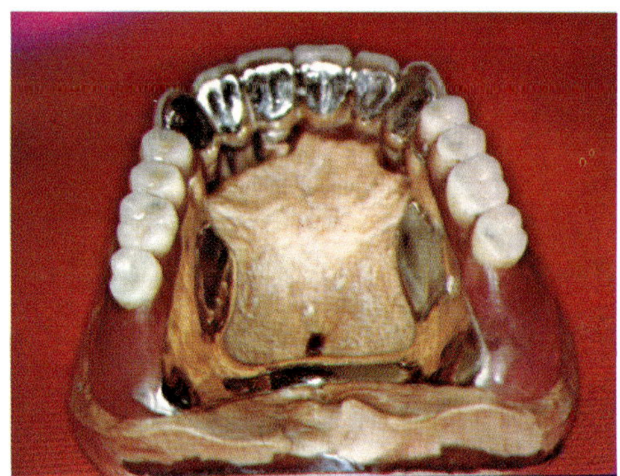

Fig. 40-41

The facings are now replaced in the plaster cores (Figs. 40-37 and 40-38) and attached to the polished metal frame (Fig. 40-39) with poured pink wax (Fig. 40-40). The denture is now technically finished, although the teeth are only fitted to the metal frame with wax (Fig. 40-41). The denture is tried in the mouth and if all is satisfactory it is flasked.

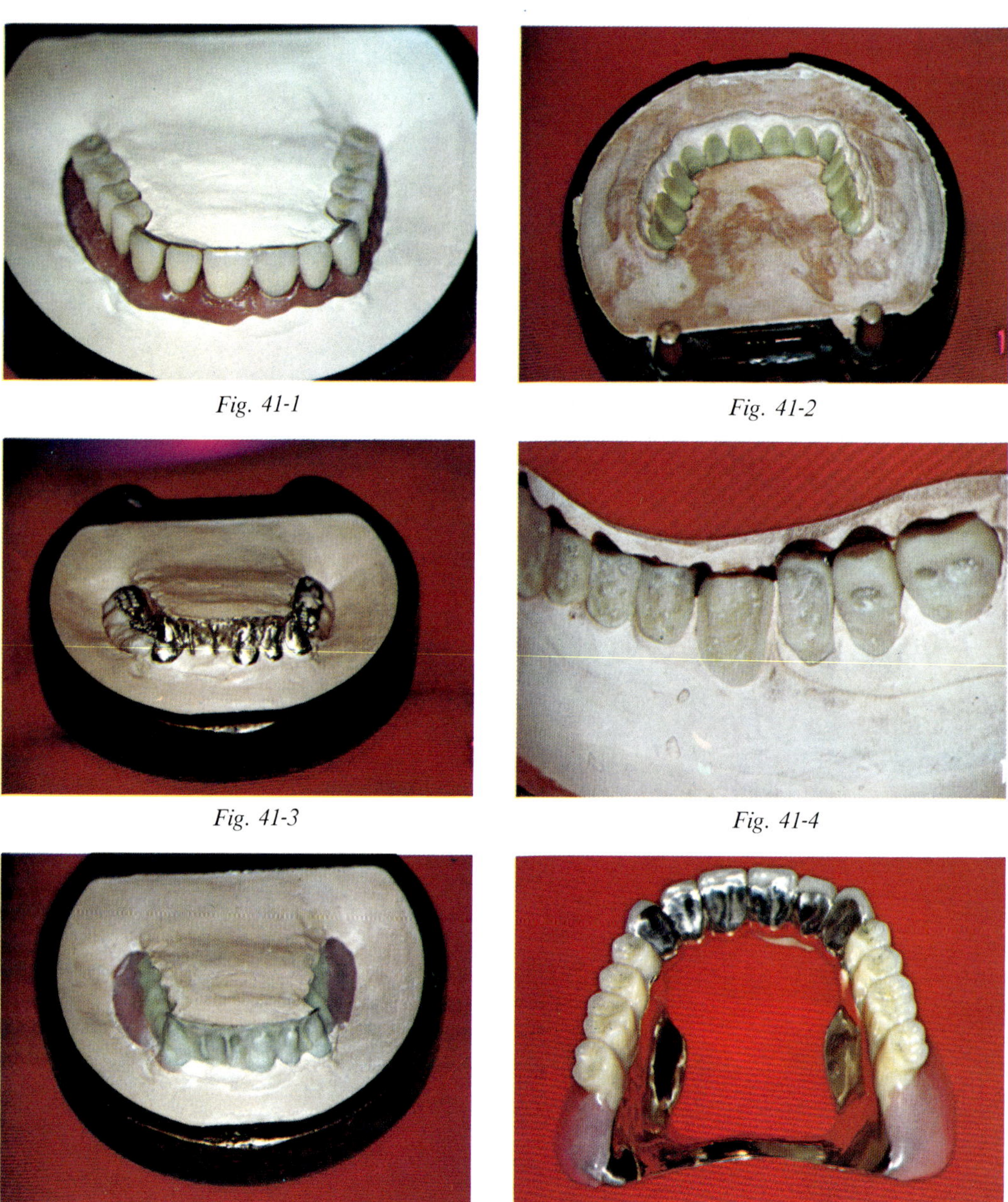

Fig. 41-1

Fig. 41-2

Fig. 41-3

Fig. 41-4

Fig. 41-5

Fig. 41-6

41. Flasking and Polishing

In my technique for flasking the denture is set in plaster (Fig. 41-1). When the flask is opened (Fig. 41-2) the facings present on one side with the metal frame on the other (Fig. 41-3). We remove the facings individually from the flask and boil them until they are absolutely wax-free. We make small grooves at the base of each facing using a very fine bur (Fig. 41-4). This ensures a firmer hold when the facings are attached to the metal frame with resin. The facings are replaced in the flask, which must be done very precisely to ensure that there are no intervening pieces of plaster between the facings and the frame. Self-curing resin is *never* used. Opaque material is used on the metal frame prior to packing. It is my policy to use Huelon color-matched resin. Simultaneously we prepare pink Huelon resin, which ultimately covers the gums. The white resin is introduced, part on the metal frame and part on the contact side of the facings (Fig. 41-5). A cellophane sheet is now positioned between the two halves of the flask. The flask is closed and slowly pressed until metal-to-metal contact of both halves of the flask is achieved. All excess resin is trimmed and a check is made that the different colored resins have not flowed into one another. The denture is cured for eight hours at 165° F. in a curing unit. The flask is removed from the curing unit, and bench cooled for 30 minutes and then cooled a further 30 minutes under cold running water. The denture is then deflasked with a great deal of care, sandpapered and polished (Fig. 41-6).

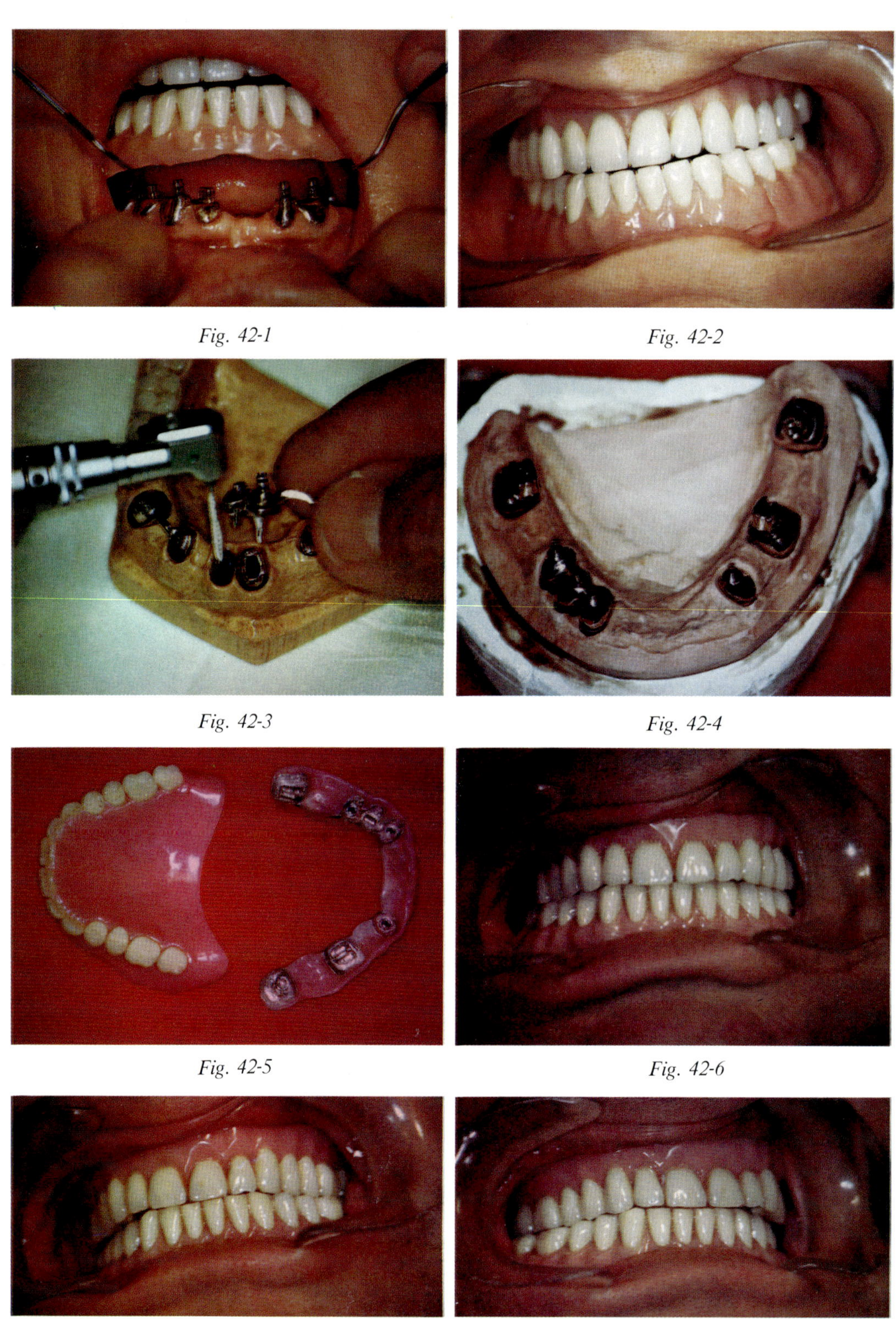

Fig. 42-1

Fig. 42-2

Fig. 42-3

Fig. 42-4

Fig. 42-5

Fig. 42-6

Fig. 42-7

Fig. 42-8

42. Cementing

The completed denture is fitted in the mouth without cementing the male parts into the roots (Fig. 42-1) and left *in situ* for 48 hours (Fig. 42-2). Antibiotic ointment is introduced into the root canals before this trial fitting. After 48 hours the denture is checked for three-point contact. If the patient is comfortable the male attachments are cemented in position with Fleck's cement (Fig. 42-3). The dentures are now inserted over the attachments in the mouth. The use of Alu-wax permits us to recheck and adjust the occlusion, with particular reference to three-point contact. After three months the articulating surfaces of the bicuspids and molars are replaced with gold if the denture has been made with plastic teeth. (Note: It is not always possible to use porcelain on the posterior teeth due to insufficient space.) We now have a lower anchored denture against a full upper denture (Figs. 15-4 to 15-8).

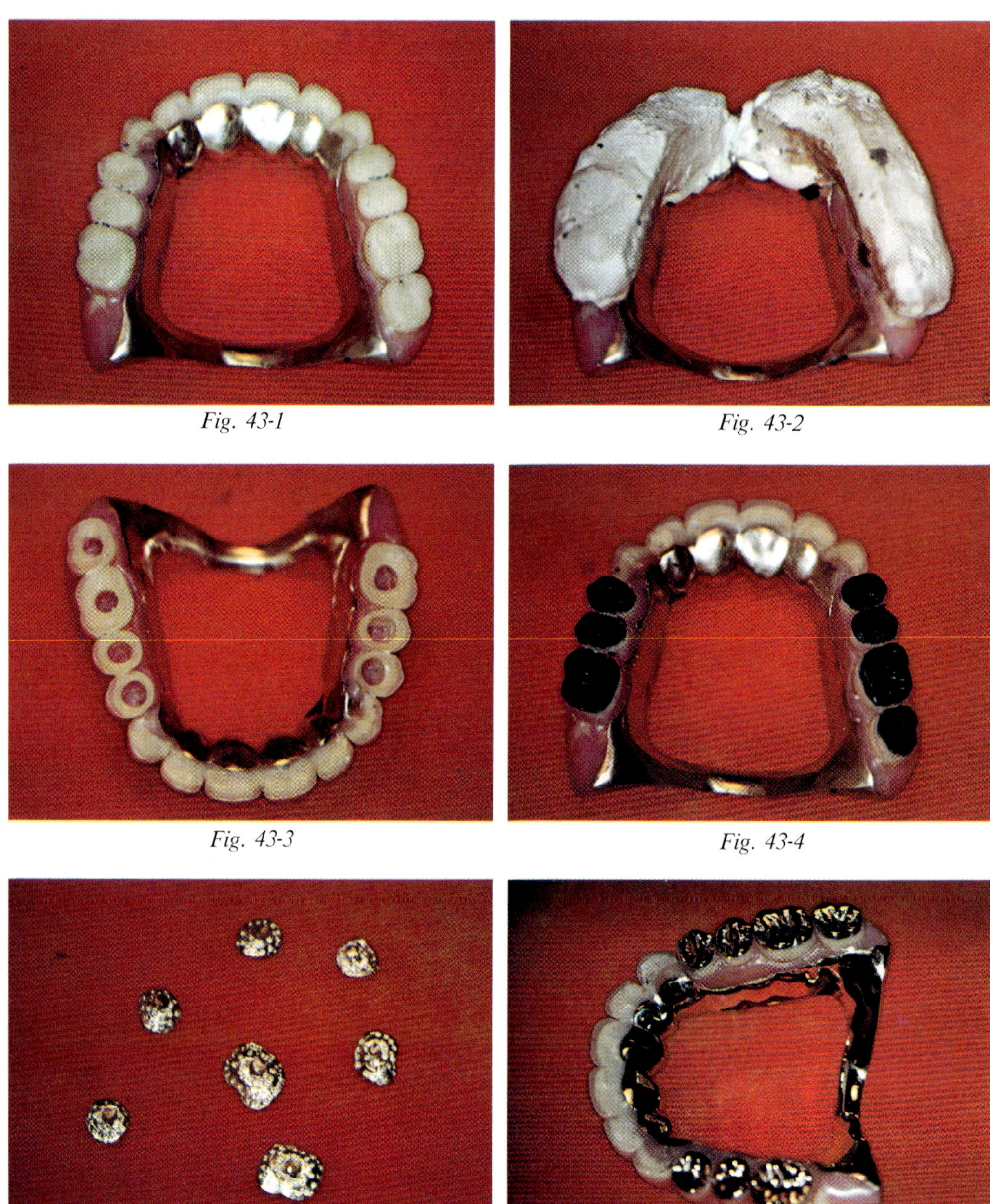

Fig. 43-1

Fig. 43-2

Fig. 43-3

Fig. 43-4

Fig. 43-5

Fig. 43-6

43. Technique for Transforming the Occlusal Surfaces of the Plastic Teeth into Gold Cusps

The technique is the same whether for the upper or lower jaw. The denture is removed from the patient's mouth (Fig. 43-1). Stone cores are made of the worn occlusal surfaces (Fig. 43-2). These acrylic teeth are prepared to receive occlusal inlays (Fig. 43-3). A wax-up over these surfaces is made using the original cores (Fig. 43-4). The blue inlay wax is then placed over the acrylic preparations. The core having been previously lubricated with petrolatum or oil, is pressed over the soft inlay wax and the occlusion refined. This wax carving is now sprued and removed from the occlusal surfaces and invested and cast. Since these castings (Fig. 43-5) have retention areas they are cemented to the acrylic teeth with self-curing resin (Fig. 43-6). The anchored denture is now completed and the occlusion is rechecked. The patient is reinstructed on denture and mouth care and requested to return to the dentist's office for four to six monthly check-ups. The case is now complete.

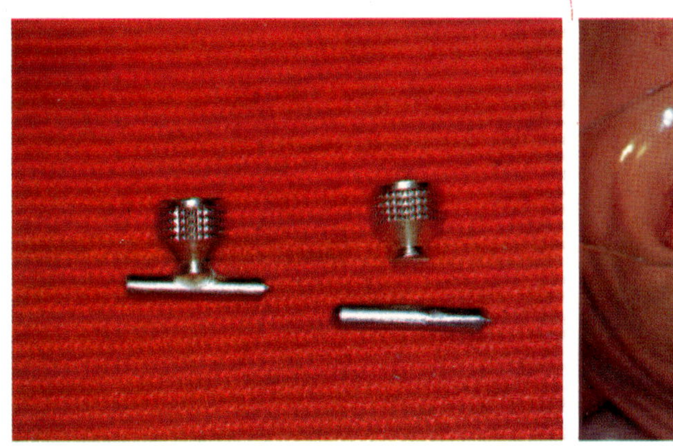

Fig. 44-1

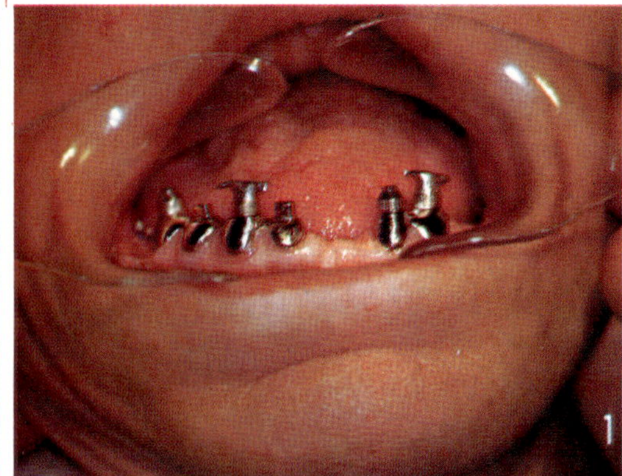

Fig. 44-2

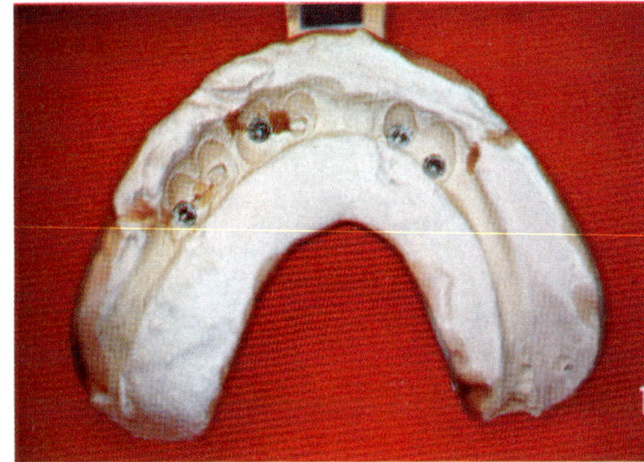

Fig. 44-3

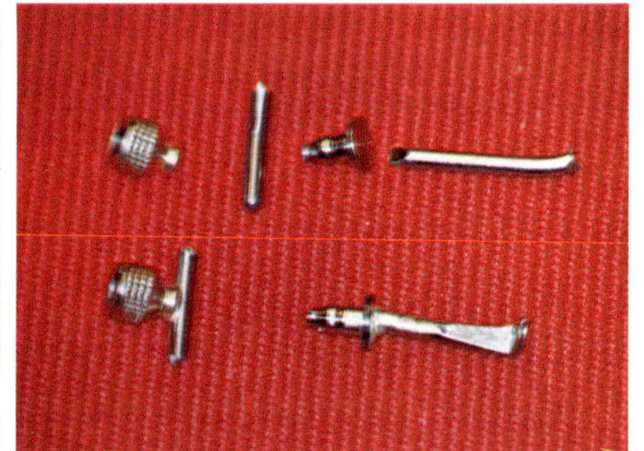

Fig. 44-4

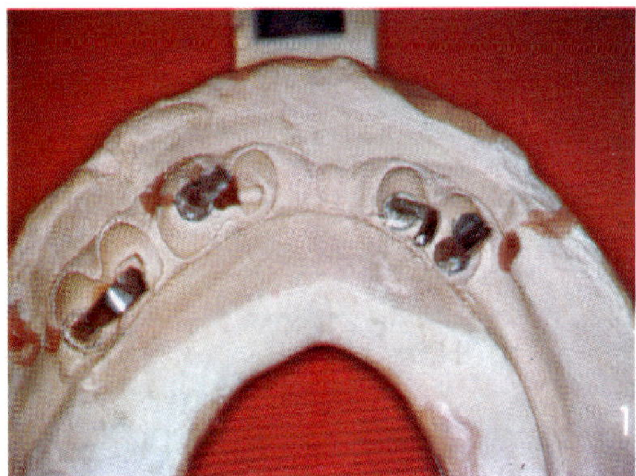

Fig. 44-5

44. Repairs

Whichever variation of prosthetic work we have completed in the mouth we may be faced at any time with the necessity for maintenance or repairs In the case of anchored dentures there are three principal categories of repair.

The metal frame

It is possible for the frame to distort or break because an insufficient thickness of gold was used by the technician, and in consequence, the frame is unable to cope with stress. If this should occur we must resolder the frame with or without an additional layer of gold at the site of the break. In order to achieve such a repair we must be able to reproduce in a plaster model the exact position of the male attachments. To do this we solder on top of several Gerber female parts a "T" bar made of gold alloy (Fig. 44-1). We remove the fractured anchored denture and place in the mouth on every male Gerber the female part with the special "T" bar top (Fig. 44-2). A plaster impression is now taken and the female attachments are retained in the impression (Fig. 44-3). We then prepare male parts by soldering a fixation pivot to the top (Fig. 44-4). The male parts are now introduced into the female parts which are still retained in the plaster model, leaving the soldered pivots protruding (Fig. 44-5). The plaster impression is now poured, and the resulting model reproduces exactly

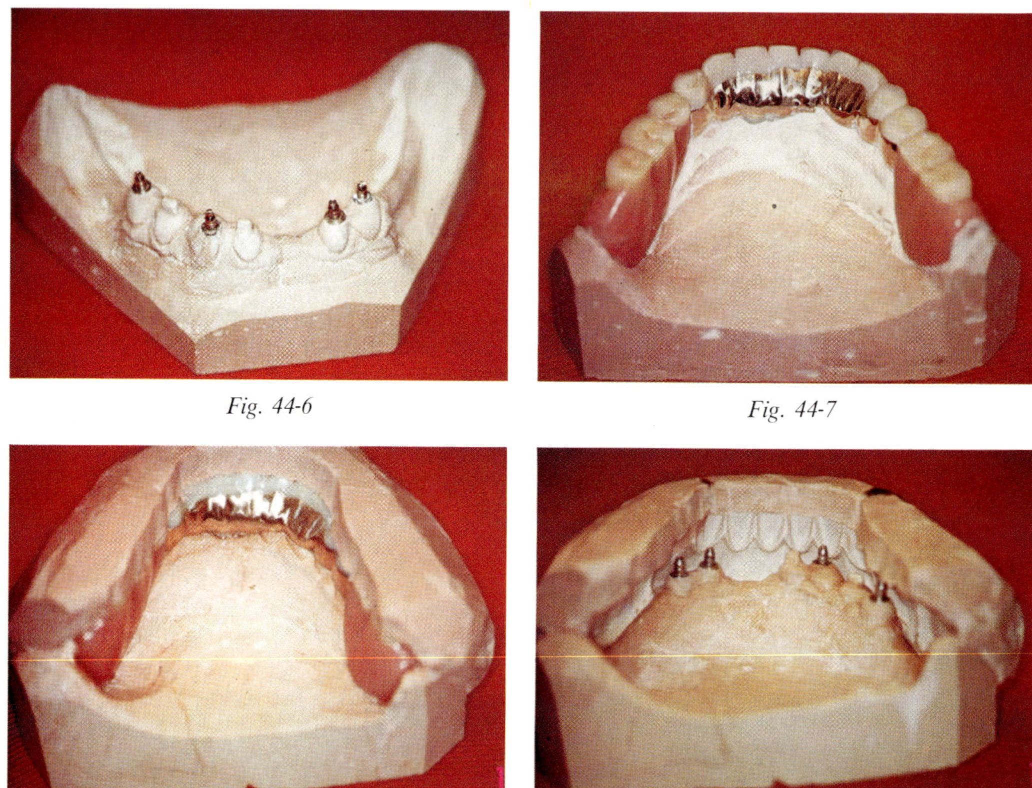

Fig. 44-6

Fig. 44-7

Fig. 44-8

Fig. 44-9

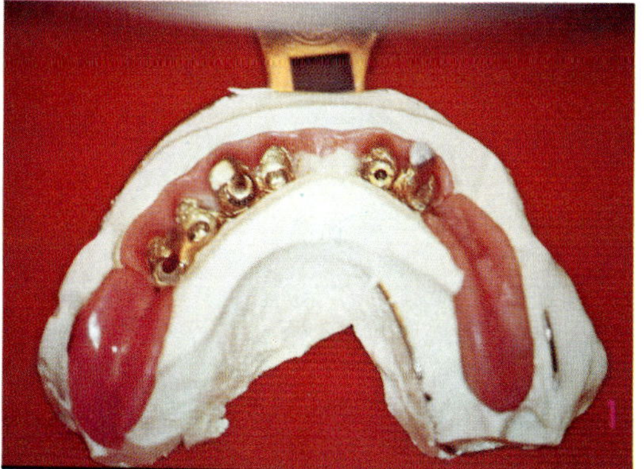

Fig. 44-10

the position of the male attachments in the mouth (Fig. 44-6). We then position the fractured denture on the model (Fig. 44-7) and take plaster cores (Fig. 44-8). Once in possession of the plaster cores (Fig. 44-9), all the teeth and facings are removed from the frame using a very fine round bur mounted on a hand piece. All the resin used to fix the teeth and facings to the frame is removed. Grooves are made on the facings as if we were building a new denture. Any remaining resin on the frame is burnt out, leaving us with a resin-free frame. The broken parts of the frame are repositioned accurately on the model and with soldering investment are held in their correct position. (Because this soldering procedure is a routine in prosthetic dentistry I shall not enlarge upon it further.) Once the frame is soldered we reposition it on the model, and if all procedures have been correctly done the fit is faultless. The frame is now tried in the mouth as an extra precaution. We complete the denture—attaching facings, curing, polishing, and so on—as described for the original denture.

Facings and teeth

If the retention in the facings and teeth is inadequate they will fall off with continued wear, or will break (Fig. 41-4). In these cases an alginate impression is taken with the denture in the mouth, resulting in an impression holding the denture (Fig. 44-10). We place male attachments with pivots (as shown in the section on repairing the metal frame) in the denture (Fig. 44-5). The impression is poured, giving us the exact position of the male attachments on the model (Fig. 44-6). If for example only one facing needs replacing and fixing, this can be achieved with color-matched self-curing acrylic. This is a very quick repair. If repair is more extensive we must use the plaster core technique described when the original denture was built.

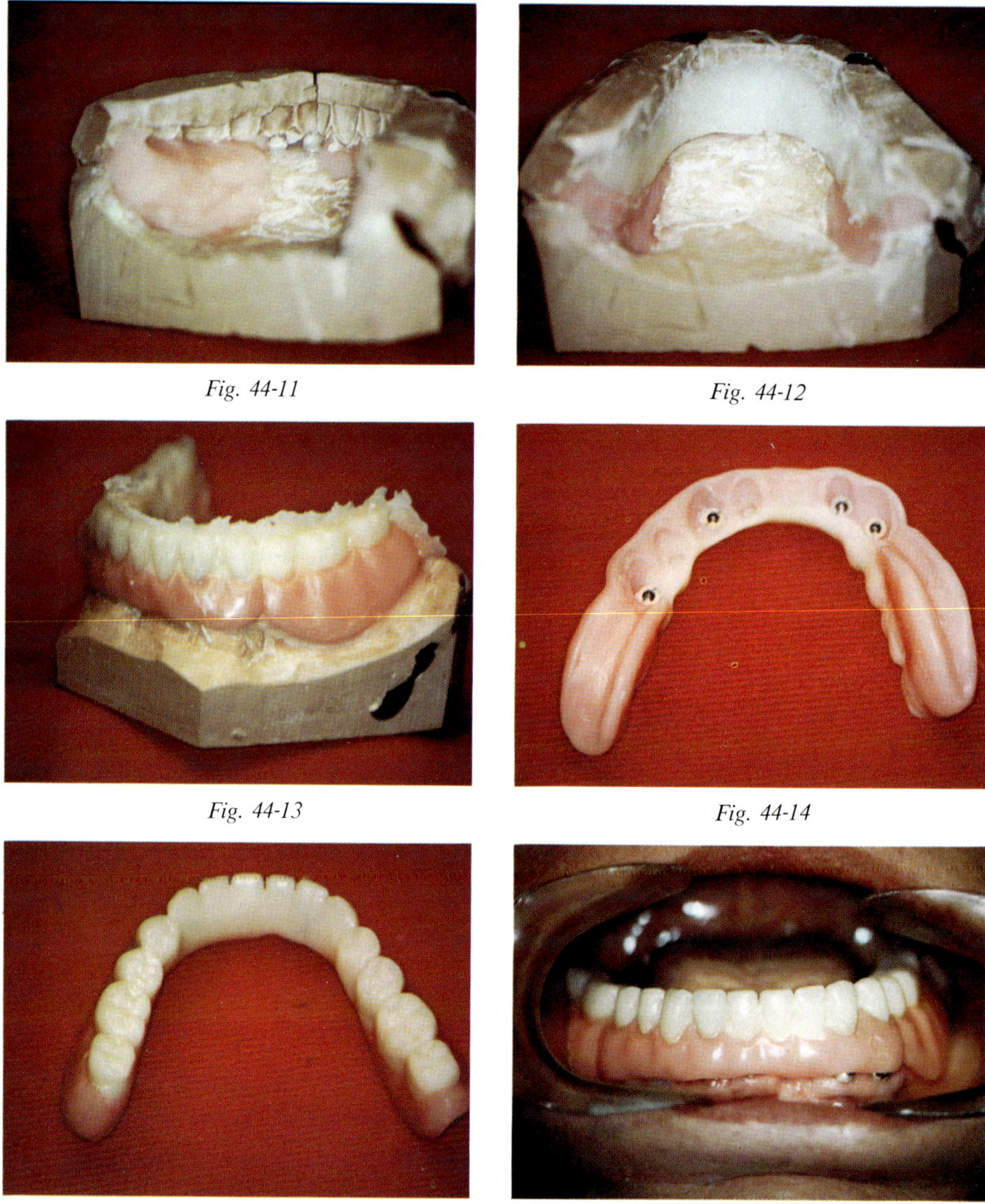

Fig. 44-11

Fig. 44-12

Fig. 44-13

Fig. 44-14

Fig. 44-15

Fig. 44-16

Since plastic facings wear with time the dentist may be faced with the problem of replacement. However, these facings are easily replaced by adapting the same technique as for broken facings.

The abutments

After many years of service any of the abutments may need to be extracted. Here now is realized the advantage of the anchored denture technique: It does not depend upon any specific number of abutments; once the abutment is extracted the denture is rebased and the patient is comfortable. Eventually he may lose—say, all the abutments on the upper jaw. The dentist will experience no difficulty in building a complete denture and obtaining three-point contact in function. Since a long laboratory procedure is involved in these repairs a temporary anchored denture is built of resin. Thus, for a few days while the new denture is being made the patient is comfortable with the temporary denture.

Technique for duplicating the anchored denture in resin

As has been previously described, we are in possession of a plaster model reproducing the mouth on which we are going to make the repairs. We are also in possession of plaster cores. Resin is poured (Figs. 44-11 and 44-12) into the space occupied by the facings and the frame. Previously we will have painted the model and plaster cores with a separating medium so that the hardened resin can easily be removed (Fig. 44-13). The anchored denture is now removed from the model, trimmed and polished (Figs. 44-14 and 44-15). It is now inserted over the male attachments in the mouth (Fig. 44-16) and the articulation rechecked.

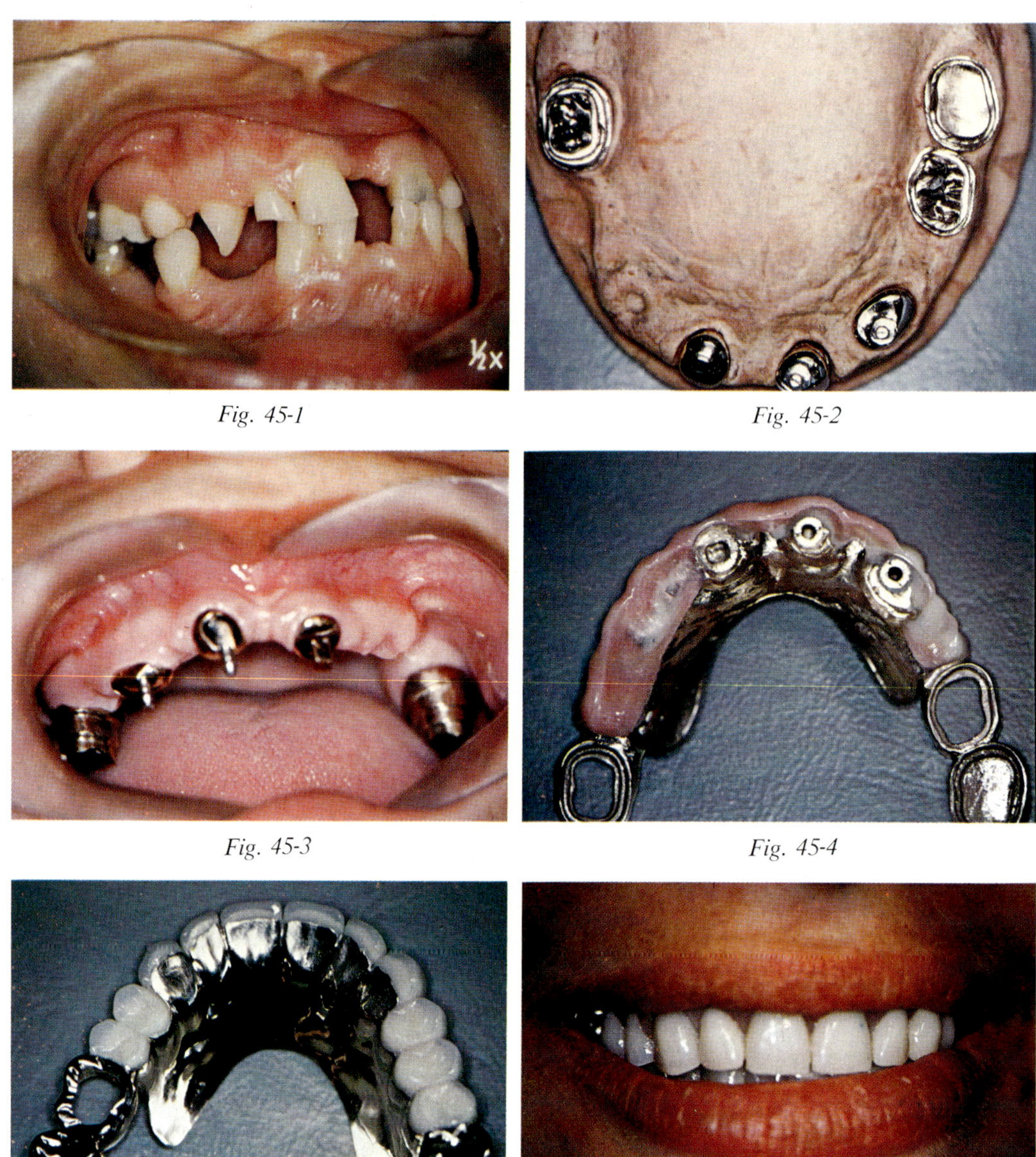

Fig. 45-1

Fig. 45-2

Fig. 45-3

Fig. 45-4

Fig. 45-5

Fig. 45-6

45. Selected Case Histories

In previous chapters we have described the techniques required for the construction of the typical anchored denture. We shall now consider variations in the use of anchored dentures, whether against natural teeth, fixed bridgework or a full denture.

Case number 1

A fifteen-year-old girl was referred to us by her dentist. She presented with a malocclusion due to partial anodontia, with both deciduous and permanent teeth in the mouth (Fig. 45-1). This case was frought with additional problems: Not only was the patient very young but she was at the time living in Cambodia with no opportunity for regular follow-up. Our primary objective was to decide which teeth could be kept and used as abutments. On the lower jaw the following teeth were retained: the two cuspids, the second bicuspids and the two second molars. As these teeth were solidly implanted and well positioned, we were able to construct a fixed 14-tooth bridge in gold and porcelain. The two molars were already devitalised teeth and the bicuspids had very large pulps. Carefully considering the age and environment of the patient I preferred to build complete crowns instead of the three quarter crowns, thus ensuring that no decay could in the future endanger her bridge.

On the upper jaw I retained five permanent teeth and one deciduous molar that I found to be solidly implanted, having undergone no root resorption. The remaining permanent teeth consisted of the two first molars, the right cuspid and the two centrals. With the remaining teeth positioned as they were it was impossible to build a fixed bridge or a partial denture that could stabilize the teeth. Therefore, an anchored denture was planned (Fig. 45-2, attachments on model; Fig. 45-3, attachments in mouth; Figs. 45-4 and 45-5, anchored denture complete).

Before we could begin to build this mouth, her temporomandibular joint dysfunction was treated with a bite plane (as previously described in the text), and as a result three-point contact was achieved with the anchored upper denture against a fixed lower bridge (Fig. 45-6, aesthetic appearance of the mouth after treatment). The application of this technique (i.e., anchored dentures in the case of partial anodontia) can also be applied for those patients with a cleft palate.

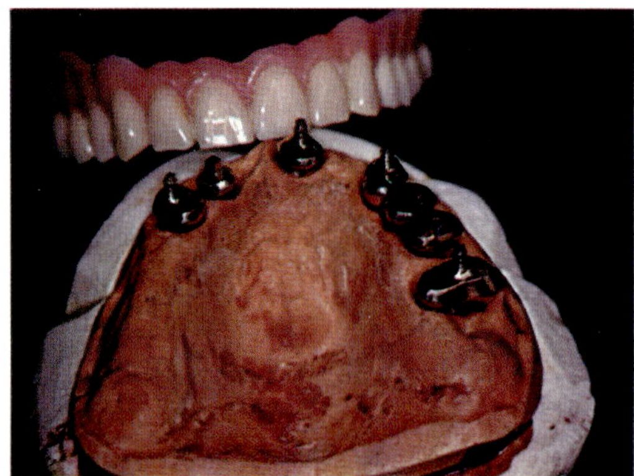

Fig. 45-7

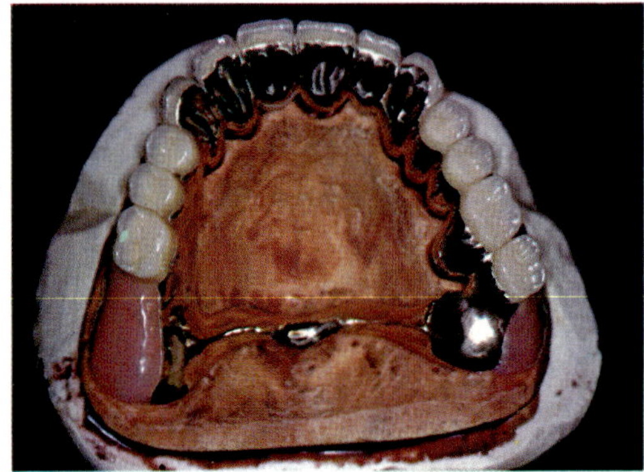

Fig. 45-8

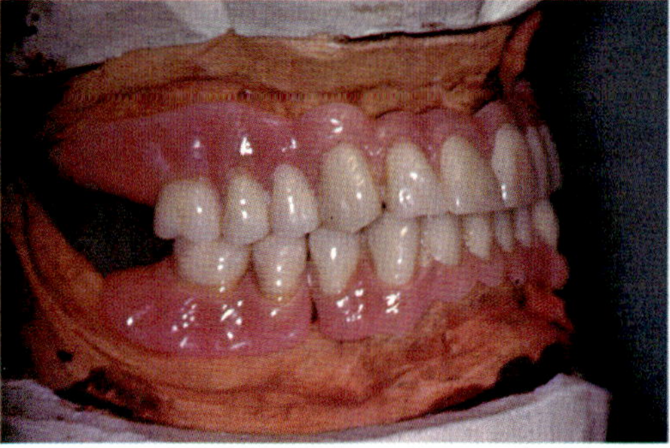

Fig. 45-9

Case number 2

A second case involving an anchored denture, particularly interesting because of the large degree of bone resorption. This is represented by the large amount of pink resin needed to build the teeth up to the correct vertical dimension (Figs. 45-7, 45-8 and 45-9).

INDEX

Numbers in italics indicate a figure, "n" following a page number indicates a footnote.